A Journey to Health:

Overcoming Inflammatory Bowel Disease

Larry K. Hartsfield, Ph.D.

This book is not intended to substitute for the advice of physicians. Readers should consult their physician regularly on issues of health.

Copyright 2011

Wolfdancer Publishing

211 Oak Drive

Durango, Colorado 81301

970-259-1812

Printed in the United States of America

1st edition

ISBN-13: 978-0-9839190-0-1

ISBN-10: 0983919003

Hartsfield, Larry K. A Journey to Health: Overcoming Inflammatory Bowel Disease Larry K. Hartsfield, Ph.D.

This book is dedicated to all those suffering from chronic diseases, but it is especially dedicated to two people:

Dr. Patrick Gerstenberger, the kind of brilliant and open-minded physician everyone should be so lucky to have—and I am.

and

Ellen, who provided the support and love to help me heal and encouraged me to write this book. Thanks for being a superb editor too.

Larry K Hartsfield

Contents

Chapter 1: Ulcerative Colitis: My Experience 1
Chapter 2: Defining Inflammatory Bowel Disease: Ulcerative Colitis and Crohn's Disease. 24
Chapter 3: Diet: Standard Approaches and Some Alternatives. . . 34
Chapter 4: I Am Not a Disease. 44
Chapter 5: The Ecology of Illness: An Ecological Perspective. . . 46
Chapter 6: The Standard American Carbohydrate-Based Diet and the Diseases of Civilization. 60
Chapter 7: Carrageenan: A Major Villain. 76
Chapter 8: The Fiber Problem. 81
Chapter 9: Sugar and Sweeteners. 89
Chapter 10: Soy. 93
Chapter 11: Cereal Grains, Gluten, and the Specific Carbohydrate Diet. 99
Chapter 12: Alternative Approaches to Treating Inflammatory Bowel Disease. 105
Chapter 13: Vitamins and Supplements. 109
Chapter 14: My Version of a Diet for Inflammatory Bowel Disease: Keeping It Simple. 112
Chapter 15: Growing a Healthy Mind. 116
Chapter 16: Revisioning Illness. 122
Chapter 17: Readings and Sources. 127

Disclaimer

As you read this book, please remember that I am not a medical doctor. I am a professor of English and Environmental Studies, and I have tried to bring an environmental and ecological perspective to this book—a perspective which stresses systems and how systems work rather than a narrow focus on one part of a system. This is an account of how I have healed from chronic inflammatory bowel disease. These are things that have worked for me. If you choose to follow some of the suggestions I offer in this book, please do so under the care and guidance of your physician. Under no circumstances should you stop taking your prescribed medications unless your doctor agrees. The information in this book contains my observations and is based only on my experience and my interpretation of the reading and research I've done.

Chapter 1
Ulcerative Colitis: My Experience

All of my training as an academic and professor urges me to "be objective" and keep myself out of my writing. I'm a private person and sometimes find it hard to share. In spite of those obstacles, I'm willing to write about my experiences with this illness in the hope that this story may help others avoid the misery I endured and that I know many readers are coping with on a daily basis. This is an account of my experience and of what has worked for me, the story of my journey to wellness and to a point where I consider myself "cured" of ulcerative colitis. Perhaps something here will also be useful to you. I know the conventional medical wisdom is that this is a chronic disease that one has to live with for the rest of one's life. However, I've now lived more than five years without a flare and have never felt healthier. My energy is restored, and I live with no symptoms of ulcerative colitis or any complications. Some of what I have to say will be controversial, and some of this material will challenge the medical, pharmaceutical, and nutritionist establishments. Through a huge amount of trial and error, experimentation and close observation, extensive reading and research, and support from an open-minded and well-informed gastroenterologist who was willing to support my explorations, I've discovered things that have and have not worked for me. Please take what is useful to you and leave the rest behind. Always, someone with an illness needs to be under a physician's care and should not change current medications or undertake new approaches without a physician's guidance, supervision, and support. I do believe I have been able to put information together from different sources in a way that is missing from traditional medical approaches to Inflammatory Bowel Disease, and I hope that this book will help others avoid much of the pain and distress that often accompany this cluster of auto-immune diseases. If this book helps even one person overcome Inflammatory Bowel Disease, then the labor involved in writing this book will have been well worth it.

My real problems began in the summer of 1992 when I returned from a month-long period of teaching in Japan. I was then 39 years old, and I had spent a week in Tokyo, then three weeks at a remote (yes, I know it's population-dense Japan, but there are still some pretty isolated areas) resort area on the shores of Lake Saiko near Mount Fuji. It had been a hard month with long days and little sleep as I helped prepare 35 Japanese students for their move to the United States where they would attend college. The food had been abysmal at this "resort," there was no place within walking distance to get anything else to eat, and I was eating a lot of soy and seaweed. I had also bummed some smokes after several years without tobacco, but stopped smoking completely when I left Japan in June.

A few days after I returned home, I started experiencing diarrhea, which before long had turned into bloody diarrhea. In no time I was making 10 to 20 trips to the toilet each day, experiencing severe urgency, and losing weight. I went to my GP and the diagnosis nightmare (with which many of you are familiar) began. The first thought was that I had picked up some sort of amoeba or other parasite in Japan. After all of those tests were negative, we tried testing for Giardia. Negative again. The tests continued and eventually, in August of 1992, my GP sent me to a gastroenterologist. He listened to my story and immediately did a sigmoidoscopy in his office. A few minutes later he told me I had ulcerative proctitis. I had never even heard of this disease and had no idea what it was. He was a patient man and spent about 30 minutes explaining to me that I had a chronic disease, ulcerative colitis, which I would have to live with for the rest of my life. I was lucky because it was confined to my rectum and the lower part of the large intestine and perhaps it wouldn't spread beyond that area. He told me that the specific kind of ulcerative colitis I had was ulcerative proctitis because it was confined to the lower area of the colon.

I didn't even know what autoimmune diseases were, so he explained these to me as well. He assured me that the best medical evidence indicated that neither diet nor stress had anything much to do with this disease. The illness probably had a genetic component, but much of the etiology of the disease was a mystery. He did tell me to keep an eye out for foods that seemed to bother me or to make the symptoms worse and to avoid those. He also recommended that I avoid whole milk products. He explained the treatment options to me, but told me that almost all patients could be treated successfully with sulfasalazine. I also learned that this disease would increase my risk of colon cancer, and that after I turned 50, I would have to have yearly colonoscopies. A good friend had just died from colon cancer, so this didn't do great things for my spirits. Since the disease was confined to the very end of my colon, my doctor's first suggestion was that we try sulfasalazine suppositories and fiber. I left his office with a prescription for the suppository and an appointment two weeks later to check on my progress.

I'm sure those with this illness can remember when you were diagnosed. I left his office depressed, confused, and worried. I had just remarried, and I was responsible for my three children. How was I going to continue a heavy work schedule, maintain my parenting responsibilities, and keep things right in a new marriage?

Looking back at this time now, I'm astonished at how quickly and easily I slid into one of the worst stances toward this disease that I could have adopted. I decided that I was going to have this disease forever. This disease was going to change everything about my life and everything in my life. I was no longer the person I thought I was—an active cyclist, hiker, skier, photographer who spent much of my time outdoors or involved with environmental groups and causes. Within hours I allowed the diagnosis and the disease to define me, and I allowed the disease to become the central fact in my life. This was real. This was not going to disappear. I needed to start finding ways to deal with this new trajectory for my life.

I didn't have the heart to tell my children immediately. I filled the prescription and noticed some minimal improvement in my symptoms. I also began researching ulcerative colitis, Crohn's disease, and autoimmune diseases. I'm an academic, and research is how I had learned to bring order and perspective to my world. Two weeks later I returned to the gastroenterologist, had another sigmoidoscopy, and a blood draw. This initial flare resolved itself pretty quickly, and I was able to stop using the suppositories although I continued with the daily fiber.

I did pretty well until February of 1993 (six months later) when another flare began. Suddenly I was going to the bathroom 20 to 30 times a day and seeing quite a bit of blood in the toilet. I saw my gastroenterologist and had some blood tests which revealed that I was also anemic. I left his office with a prescription for sulfasalazine and instructions that I should avoid too much sun exposure since the sulfasalazine could cause sun sensitivity. Both the ulcerative colitis and the anemia seemed to resolve themselves. Another flare started in May of 1993 after I took the NSAID (non-steroidal anti-flammatory drugs) medication Anaprox for lower back pain. In August the results of a blood test revealed that my white blood cell count was dangerously low—a condition called leukopenia. I saw the gastroenterologist in early September and found that I apparently could not metabolize sulfasalazine because of the way it interacted with my bone marrow and the production of white blood cells. I also found out that the ulcerative proctitis had become full-blown ulcerative colitis although it seemed to be confined to the left side of my colon. We discussed the negatives of NSAIDS (which should never be used by a person suffering from Inflammatory Bowel Disease) and my former tobacco use and its possible relation to ulcerative colitis. This time I left with a prescription for olsalazine (a way of getting the salazine to my intestines that avoided the sulfa). He also told me to discontinue the fiber since that wasn't good for ulcerative colitis although it could be useful when the disease was confined to the rectum—the way my ulcerative colitis had originally presented.

My symptoms didn't improve and neither did the low white blood count. In early October he took me off the olsalazine and decided to try another delivery system, mesalimine, as well as metronidazole, an antibiotic. I also restarted the salazine enemas. Unfortunately I subsequently had the same issues with mesalamine, and my symptoms weren't improving. Nothing had improved by the end of October. I felt like I had been shitting myself to death for months now. At the end of October we reviewed my treatment options. These included continuing the enemas and adding corticosteroid therapy.

Prior to this late October appointment I had taken a careful look back at my earlier life, and I remembered that I had bled rectally years ago when I had stopped smoking in 1975 and that the blood had disappeared after I started smoking again. When I quit smoking for good in 1981, I didn't see any gastric symptoms, but I developed severe lower back pain. At the time I blamed it on stress. Now I know that this lower back pain can also be a symptom of ulcerative colitis. As a result, I spent the 1970s and 1980s periodically taking aspirin, ibuprofen, and prescription pain medications (including NSAIDs) for this pain. I believe these drugs may have contributed to the development of full-blown ulcerative colitis. Could there be a connection between smoking and this disease? On this visit to the gastroenterologist I asked him about this, and, to my surprise, he said that there was a connection. Ex-smokers tended to develop ulcerative colitis at a higher rate than non-smokers and there was some evidence that nicotine provided protection against ulcerative colitis. He also showed me an article that reported some success treating ulcerative colitis with transdermal nicotine patches. He did not recommend that I start smoking, although it was clear that he was also getting frustrated at my failure to respond positively to medication. He wanted to try prednisone, but after he explained the extensive potential side effects, I declined the steroid treatment. I decided to try the transdermal nicotine patches since I had already been wondering about a connection between smoking and ulcerative colitis. I was on sabbatical that fall to try to finish a book (which still isn't finished) and although I was making progress on the book, the medical issues were interfering with my research, my writing, and with every other aspect of my life.

Unfortunately the patches didn't bring the symptoms into remission, and in mid-November I decided to try smoking to see if that made a difference. I saw the gastroenterologist again in early December, and he recommended that I stop smoking and go back to the patches at a higher dose of nicotine. I was seeing some relief of symptoms with the smoking, so I didn't make this switch back to the patches. We determined that because of the toxic effects of 5-ASA (salazine) drugs on my bone marrow that I would discontinue all forms of these immediately and not use them in the future. By January of 1994 my symptoms were in complete remission. I met with my gastroenterologist in February of 1994, and he supported my decision to start smoking as therapy and suggested that five to seven cigarettes a day were probably safer than long-term corticosteroid use. A colonoscopy in December of 1996 showed that the ulcerative colitis was in complete remission, and the gastroenterologist reaffirmed that this seemed a reasonable approach to managing the disease as opposed to long-term steroid use.

When I look at the past with the knowledge I have now, I realize that I probably had my first bout with ulcerative colitis in 1975 when I was 22 years old. I was a graduate student, and my first child had just been born—lots of stress. I quit smoking at his birth and about a month later started experiencing pretty severe bleeding from my rectum. I went to the doctor in a small southern Illinois town who told me it was a hemorrhoid and recommended that I sit in a hot bath several times a day. I started smoking again, the blood disappeared, and I didn't worry about it. I stopped smoking for good when my third child was born in 1981. I was near the completion of my dissertation and Ph.D., and it seemed like a good time to quit. I didn't start bleeding again, but I did have bouts of severe lower back pain over the next 10 years. For months at a time I needed help getting in and out of bed and at times used a walking stick. I was in my thirties, and that seemed far too young for me to be physically "falling apart."

I also had an episode that I'm sure was UC related in the mid-80s. I visited an ophthalmologist for my annual eye exam who sent me to see my GP. I had no concept of ulcerative colitis at this time, but my physician ran a number of tests on me and finally told me that the ophthalmologist had detected some issues in my eye that he thought might indicate I had leukemia. It turned out that I didn't have cancer, and the only thing that was showing up in the battery of tests was some protein in my urine. Eventually a kidney specialist diagnosed me with nonspecific membranous nephritis. Was this problem another symptom of IBD? I don't know, but my guess is that it was.

Although smoking kept the ulcerative colitis in complete remission, I was very unhappy about the smoking and felt like I was setting a bad example for my children, which bothered me deeply. I also thought I was setting a bad example for my students. In addition to these issues, I was also active in local environmental causes—how could I be environmentally conscious and smoke? I had bought into the anti-smoking attitude that suggests that smoking contributes to the pollution not only of our bodies but of the larger community. I felt like I was doing something immoral, something bad, something unethical. Just short of four years after starting to smoke, I stopped smoking in January 1998 even though I had been in complete remission for those last four years. I managed to go about seven months before an ulcerative colitis flare took off. This flare was probably triggered by antibiotics. I took the antibiotic Cephalexin in June and July for an infected salivary gland and then for folliculitis. Of course, I should have asked why I suddenly started getting these infections, but I didn't. I still hadn't taken a stance in which I shared full responsibility for my health. I began to notice changes in my bowels in late July. I knew that antibiotic use could damage the bacterial flora of the intestine and bring on flares, but I'd been almost four years without a flare, and I really didn't think about this before taking the antibiotic. The stress level I was experiencing also rose when my then wife and I separated in early August. After a visit to my general practitioner, I added Prozac to my medications to try to combat the depression I found myself dealing with. I never had any problems with Prozac, although it also didn't do much for the depression. For me, exercise and staying as busy as possible seemed like better solutions to depression than a drug, so I went off of the Prozac after a few months. I've read some studies that suggest Prozac or other anti-depressants might be helpful in treating flares of Inflammatory Bowel Disease, and I know one person who claims that it helps keep her in remission. This wasn't my experience, but it might work for some people.

Soon I was in a full-blown flare and heading to the toilet fifteen to twenty-five times a day to watch the toilet bowl fill with blood. I've had a number of extreme flares. In the books about IBD that I've read, physicians and other authors talk about severe cases of ulcerative colitis with 10 to 20 trips to the bathroom a day. Mine tended to be 20-30 trips to the bathroom daily with lots of blood, urgency, and all of the other symptoms of severe ulcerative colitis. I had to start keeping extra underwear and pants at school, "just in case." I felt like I was on the verge of publicly humiliating myself at any moment.

I returned to my gastroenterologist, and he scheduled me for a colonoscopy. After the colonoscopy, we talked. No longer was the ulcerative colitis confined to the left side of my large intestine. The

IBD had moved throughout the entire colon. During this conversation, I told him that I did not want to start smoking again, so we decided to use the transdermal nicotine patches and give metronidazole another try. This time the patches didn't help, nor did the metronidazole, but I still did not want to start smoking again. I decided I was willing to try the corticosteroid, prednisone. He agreed, and I began with 25 mg of prednisone daily. That didn't help, so he adjusted the dosage to 50 mg daily, 40 mg in the morning and 10 mg in the evening. At this dosage, I started seeing improvements, and the gastroenterologist told me I'd be on that for a couple of weeks and then he'd have me slowly taper off of the prednisone.

The prednisone was like a miracle: my appetite returned, I had enormous amounts of energy, and I was churning out work at a high rate. I had become chair of my academic department, so the ability to work ceaselessly was a big help. Best of all, my symptoms disappeared. Things were going well until I had tapered off to about 25 mg of prednisone daily. At that point my symptoms returned, so I went back up on the higher dosage of prednisone. I hadn't had any of the more obvious side effects of prednisone during this first round—I'd gained a little weight, but that's about all. Since I was underweight, I saw this just as an added benefit. I eventually tapered off the prednisone, but began using hydrocortisone suppositories to maintain the remission.

Even with the hydrocortisone suppositories I wasn't able to maintain remission, and in early February 1999 another flare started which was confirmed by a colonoscopy. The ulcerative colitis had now spread throughout my colon, and my diagnosis became chronic ulcerative pancolitis. In March I was back to forty mg of prednisone a day, and I began taking 50 mg daily of the immunomodulator 6-mercaptopurine (6mp). I had some real questions about taking 6mp because of potential side effects such as lymphoma and the potential spontaneous abortions if a sexual partner became pregnant. Also, 6mp is generally considered a kind of chemotherapy drug, and that scared me as well. The thought of being on a kind of chemotherapy when I didn't even have cancer was of grave concern to me. On the other hand, I was at the end of my rope, and I wasn't involved with anyone. Still, hearing about the side effects of this drug sent me into a tailspin. I truly felt like I had lost control of my body, of myself. I didn't make an immediate decision, but he gave me the names of a couple of patients who were on 6mp and suggested I talk to them.

I did, and after these conversations with sympathetic and understanding fellow-sufferers, I decided to start the 6mp. This was going to mean I had to avoid alcohol completely (not a problem) and have frequent blood tests to see how I tolerated the 6mp. I hated having my blood drawn, but the alternatives seemed worse. Bit by bit this disease seemed to be destroying my old self and replacing it with a new identity—that of a sick person whose illness was becoming fundamental to his identity. Ulcerative colitis had become the central defining fact in my life.

By May I had been on the 6mp for two months but was still taking 20 mg of prednisone daily, which continued until August when I was able to maintain remission until February of 2000. The 6mp seemed to work pretty well although I would have a flare every time I found myself facing stress. The next few years did, unfortunately, contain a lot of stress—some of it work-related as I chaired a large department, some of it family-related. I seemed to settle into a pattern of two-three flares a year. Some of the flares were major and some were relatively minor, but all involved bleeding, mucus, urgency and numerous trips to the bathroom. Most of them came under control with some prednisone and the 6mp, which I had been taking without a break since starting it. I learned to live with this unwelcome co-inhabiter of my body—I tried to deal with the disease when it flared and otherwise tried not to think about it (although it was always present in one way or another in my mind). I simply accepted that this was a chronic condition I would live with for the rest of my life and did my best to "manage" the disease.

I met Ellen in December of 1999 at a dance, which is truly ironic to anyone who knows me. Our connection was immediate, and even though I dreaded doing so, I told her about the ulcerative colitis very early in our relationship. She had lost her first husband at the age of 32, and I worried that she might not want to get involved with someone who had a chronic illness. Luckily, she was (and has always been) incredibly supportive. Ellen wanted to have children, and I began to worry about the 6mp and its potential side effects. On the other hand, I didn't really see any alternative to continuing the medication.

One of the elements of this disease that isn't often discussed is that of self-loathing, of looking at ourselves, our bodies, as objects of disgust, of horror, as things that have escaped our control and become something not only alien but sickening and unlovable. I dreaded the conversation with Ellen. If I couldn't love myself, how could anyone else love me? How could I bring another person into this nightmare? Still, I knew the conversation had to take place. One of the great blessings for my life was that she accepted me and the disease I suffered from. I prefaced the discussion by telling her that I had a "really disgusting chronic disease" that she needed to know about. She looked a bit taken aback and asked what it was. I told her, and the relief was clear. Later she told me that she thought I had been going to tell her I had a serious sexually-transmitted disease and was actually relieved.

In January of 2000 another flare started, and I went back on 30 mg of prednisone a day and increased the 6mp to 75 mg daily. A June 2000 colonoscopy showed active colitis. Eventually that flare subsided.

The path this time around was supposed to be that I would taper off the prednisone again and when I reached 30 mg per day add prednisone enemas to help me get off the oral prednisone, but this time I had an ugly surprise. I started losing my vision. Vision is central to my job and to my core sense of who I am. If I lost my ability to read, I thought, I would lose myself. Plus, vision is a handy sense to have. This symptom scared me so much that I kept it to myself except for complaining about blurry vision to my family. The fear was more concrete because I had worked with a colleague who had Crohn's for a number of years until he took medical retirement. His office was next door to mine, and I had watched the disease and the medications (mostly prednisone) literally destroy him. He deteriorated from a man who had attended college on a basketball scholarship and was happily married, to a man who had a bitter divorce, had poor relationships with his children, used two canes to walk, and became blind. In June I had another colonoscopy which revealed continuing active colitis.

Ellen and I were married in August of 2000 and after a wonderful honeymoon in Greece to meet some of her family, returned to Durango. Ellen had recently been hired to teach French at the same college where I taught and things seemed to be going as smoothly as possible. Even the ulcerative colitis was quiet. Work was difficult, though. I was elected to serve a third term as Chair of my department, but there were some difficult personnel issues, and I started having severe pain in my neck and back.

In November of 2000, I went to see my general practitioner, but he wasn't available, so I saw his physician's assistant instead and described the pain I was experiencing. She wanted me to try Vioxx to reduce the inflammation and pain. If you learn nothing else from my experience, take this lesson away: stand up for yourself when something is being prescribed for you. If you have any doubts about the medication, stand firm. I told her several times that I shouldn't take Vioxx because I had had bad experiences with aspirin, ibuprofen, and NSAIDs in the past due to my ulcerative colitis. These drugs had caused bleeding and flares for me, so I avoided them. She insisted that Vioxx, although an NSAID, was an exception and worked in a way that was different from other NSAIDs. She also insisted that this should have no impact on ulcerative colitis. Just writing this makes me pissed off—both at her and at myself. I should have stood my ground. I didn't. She gave me samples, sent me home, and I started the Vioxx in late November. Vioxx very literally almost killed me.

Two days later, Thanksgiving Day, 2000, I awoke to bloody diarrhea and mucus and the beginning of what turned out to be the worst flare I had ever experienced to that point. I blame this completely on the Vioxx, which has since been removed from the market after lawsuits, a lot of bad press, and thousands of reported deaths linked to the drug.

Once more I was on huge doses of prednisone, this time 60 mg daily, along with the 6mp, and now the blurred vision started immediately and was worse than what I had experienced before. I was afraid to drive, and I couldn't read—I thought the worst was taking place. I made an appointment with my eye doctor and finally received the answer to the problem with my vision. As I suspected, this difficulty with my vision was prednisone-related. The prednisone (he thought) had increased the sugar in my blood and was clogging the capillaries feeding my eye and causing the blurriness. As I tapered off the prednisone, my vision should improve. This had been my experience in the past, so I didn't worry about it too much. By early January of 2001 I had tapered down to 20 mg of prednisone daily but was taking 100 mg of 6mp each day. As I reduced the prednisone, the flare reasserted itself and in February I went back to 60 mg of prednisone while maintaining a 100 mg daily dose of 6mp. Once more my gastroenterologist and I discussed the possibility of a colectomy, the removal of my colon, but I was just not ready for a procedure that drastic yet.

Here's a dirty little secret. I had come to enjoy taking the prednisone. Sure, it had some horrible side effects, but I couldn't believe the energy I had. I would typically sleep from 10 pm until 1 or 1:30 am and then get up and work like a madman. I was reading an enormous number of books, researching, writing, and generally living like a meth addict without the meth.

I would, however, get tired during the day—crash severely sometimes and become a little bit disoriented. I was also thirsty all the time, and I don't mean a little thirsty—I mean thirsty as in having been in the desert for a week without fluids kind of way. I started buying bottles of apple and grape juice. I figured this was better than water since I'd be getting some nutrition and juice is one of the healthiest things we can drink, right? The more I drank, the less I slept, since I was peeing almost continuously. I also began to feel a thinness in my "self"—something that I would describe to Ellen as a feeling of "threadiness." I finally reached a point where I was sure I was going to die. This didn't bother me. I hated that I would be leaving my children and Ellen behind, but I was at peace, ready to go, and utterly without fear. I still remember sitting on the couch and recognizing that I knew I was going soon, and that I was okay with that. This was in late February of 2001.

Oddly, the next morning Ellen asked me if I could have diabetes. I thought she was crazy and asked why she would think that. She told me she had had a dream and that in the dream I had diabetes. I dismissed her concern, but the following morning when I was up at two am scouring the internet, I looked up the symptoms of diabetes. I had them all. I couldn't believe it. Surely I was too skinny to have diabetes. I called my general practitioner's office as soon as it opened, described my symptoms, and was told to cancel my classes and get to their offices immediately.

After a blood test on February 28, I found out that my blood sugar levels were 667 instead of the normal of 100-120. I was diabetic. I could have been in a coma or died at numbers lower than that. This was in early 2001 before the surge in popular awareness of and media attention to the national epidemic in diabetes. I'd been keeping most of my symptoms and discomfort to myself, and without Ellen's dream I don't think that I would have survived the month of February 2001.

I was planning to leave the next weekend to drive the 1200 miles from Durango to Olympia, Washington, where my daughter was in college, to visit her during my spring break. I told my GP that I was still going to make the trip—his response was that right now he was just trying to keep me out of the hospital, and that I would not be making this trip. It turned out that I had steroid-induced diabetes, and that my pancreas was no longer working. I started insulin injections that day, and I was given instructions on how to measure my blood sugars five times a day and on how to use insulin injections three times a day to keep my blood sugar under control. I was also immediately scheduled to see a dietician/nutritionist to discuss how to keep my blood sugar under control through diet and exercise as well as through the insulin. I learned that no one had any idea as to whether or not I would be diabetic for the rest of my life or whether my pancreas would return to normal after (if) I was off prednisone. I left having taken several more steps down the staircase of bleakness and despair about how this disease was destroying my life.

On the other hand, Ellen said, just be thankful we found out you had diabetes and can now do something about it. On March 5, 2001 I saw my gastroenterologist, and he raised the 6mp dosage to 150 mg since blood tests indicated that I apparently wasn't metabolizing the 6mp. He also told me that the ulcerative colitis had become steroid-dependent, but that it was also critical for me to avoid future courses of prednisone.

Ellen and I visited the dietician that same afternoon, and I received some advice that just didn't make sense to me. The dietician wanted me to go on a high carbohydrate diet supplemented by low-fat protein and suggested that I try to eat 13-14 servings of carbohydrates each day. I questioned the wisdom of this since I already knew that carbohydrates turn into glucose during the digestive process, and it seemed like that would only raise the blood sugar levels I was supposed to be keeping down. She insisted that this was the optimum diet for insulin-dependent diabetics, and I guess I should thank her for this because my utter disbelief caused me to finally get down to researching things for myself in depth. I can now see this as an important step on my journey to fully taking charge of my own health, but I'm still angry when I think about how many people have been given this same bad advice and have had their lives and health damaged as a result. The consumption of a diet high in carbohydrates has been linked through innumerable studies to illnesses ranging from diabetes to heart disease to the gamut of auto-immune illnesses to Alzheimer's—and that's by no means the complete list. Barry Groves, Ph.D., recommends sticking to an eating plan under 50 carbohydrates per day on most days. Christian B. Allan and Wolfgang Lutz, the authors of *Leben Ohne Brot* (*Life Without Bread* in the English edition), suggest eating about 70-75 carbohydrates a day. Dr. Richard Bernstein, in his book, *Dr. Bernstein's Diabetes Solution*, also is a proponent of a low-carbohydrate eating plan for health and longevity. The list of scholars and researchers who believe in the value of eating a low-carbohydrate diet is too long to chronicle here.

I wasn't (and still am not) ready to abandon traditional medicine, but I knew I had to take a more active role with this disease. I was scared and ready to do whatever it took to get well. My experience must parallel the experience of many other people suffering from inflammatory bowel disease. A medicine didn't work, or if it did it had such horrible side effects that in the process of controlling the malfunctions of one part of my body, other parts started malfunctioning, sometimes in ways that were more destructive than the original disease.

In many ways we're blessed today with the huge quantity of information that is readily available to us. The downside of this is that lots of bad information is also widely available to us. It's easy to search the Web and find an enormous amount of information, but how do we know what's good, what's bad, or what's being presented just to sell us one "miracle" cure or another. You can find lots of "facts" and studies on all sorts of topics, but it takes care, time, and expertise in how to evaluate sources, statistics, and what one reads to discern the good information from the sloppy, hasty, or dangerous "information." A secondary problem with searching the web is the tendency of many people to fall into hypochondria and to assume that they have the worst of all possible diseases or outcomes.

My career path has prepared me to search vast amounts of material and to apply the skills as a researcher and evaluator that I've honed throughout my professional life. My own educational background is in American Studies, an interdisciplinary field that requires its scholars to range widely through numerous disciplines such as history, literature, media studies, political science, sociology, and even medicine. In my first book I explored the professionalization of fields such as journalism, sociology, anthropology, and medicine in the late nineteenth and early twentieth centuries, so I was used to taking a "metaview" of the knowledge of a given field of study. I used these skills as a savvy researcher to find the information that would help me get better, although I never really believed at the time that I could be truly well. I just wanted to get rid of the diabetes and lead a healthier life. This book is a distillation of the advice and material that I've found useful and reputable, even though it often challenges or disagrees with the current dogma of a particular field.

The first thing I searched for was information on diabetes. I eventually ended up purchasing *Dr. Bernstein's Diabetes Solution*, and I found this book to be incredibly useful in managing the diabetes. Dr. Bernstein recommends an extremely low carbohydrate diet, and this diet helped me maintain good blood sugar levels more than any other advice I received, even though my blood sugars were still much higher than they should have been, and I had to use insulin three times a day.

Since I was having such success with diet and diabetes, I decided to do some research on diet and ulcerative colitis. In my research on diet I discovered the Specific Carbohydrate Diet. You've probably already encountered this diet if you've done much reading about inflammatory bowel disease. Today it's mentioned in a number of books, but it hadn't been mentioned in any of the books my doctor had suggested back in the early 90s, and I read everything published about ulcerative colitis when I was first diagnosed. At that time there really wasn't much available for the layperson to read, and what was available essentially followed standard medical protocols. Today the Specific Carbohydrate Diet (SCD) is mentioned or discussed in a number of books and not always in a positive way—sometimes its followers are referred to as a "cult" and generally IBD sufferers are told that they should avoid the diet because it isn't medically proven or because it's so rigorous that it's difficult to follow. I read about the diet and noticed that it shared a number of similarities with the diet Dr. Bernstein advocated, so I ordered a copy of *Breaking the Vicious Cycle*, by Elaine Gottschall. I discovered that it is indeed an extremely rigorous and limited diet, but I was ready to try it. A bit more research, and I discovered a listserv (since defunct) devoted to following the SCD. This listserv was one of the best things that happened to me. Finally I had a place to share my experiences with people suffering from the same disease and the same symptoms I knew so well. I became an active participant on the listserv and followed the diet religiously. It did help. It didn't cure me, and I no longer follow it precisely, but it did help, and some of its staples, such as homemade high-fat, lactose-free yogurt and some other recipes have become part of my family's regular diet.

  I do want to emphasize that I went on this diet only after consultation with my gastroenterologist. He was skeptical, but he didn't see how it could do any damage, so he told me to go ahead and pursue it. He also referred me to an endocrinologist to help with the diabetes. Another doctor, another round of appointments, another set of advice and directives. You've been there—you know what it's like.

  Eventually this flare tapered off. In early May I was down to 15 mg a day of prednisone, and my insulin doses were a bit lower. The endocrinologist suggested I try a new oral drug for diabetes, Avandia. My gastroenterologist said there was insufficient data on this drug and ulcerative colitis, but he would allow me to try it as long as I continued frequent blood tests.

By now both my wife and I had become experts at the Specific Carbohydrate Diet. We made all our own food when we traveled, and I could whip up a batch of almond-flour crackers at a moment's notice. We became master yogurt makers and epic yogurt eaters. As I recovered, our lives ceased to revolve around the disease so much—now they revolved around the diet. I was doing well, but I was still taking 6mp daily and using a prednisone enema every night to keep things under control. I seemed to be tapering off the prednisone successfully, but in late June my gastroenterologist called and said he was a bit concerned since my liver enzymes seemed to be raised. We left town for a four-week road trip to the East Coast in July (after a blood draw the day before leaving).

About a week later while driving through rush hour traffic in Boston, on our way to a wedding where Ellen was scheduled to be the celebrant, I received a phone call from my doctor who told me to immediately stop taking the Avandia since my liver enzymes were very high, and he was worried about the possibility of liver failure. He wanted me to come back to Durango immediately. I stopped the Avandia on his advice but decided to continue with the trip. By now I was down to 2.5 mg of prednisone daily and 100 mg of 6mp. I was also slowly weaning myself from the insulin, so my pancreas seemed to be starting to work as I tapered off the prednisone. I had another set of blood tests on July 27, and my liver enzymes were again normal, which was an enormous relief. By December of 2001 I was completely off insulin and prednisone and taking only 100mg of 6mp daily.

As I felt better, I left the SCD slowly behind and then the pattern of the disease reasserted itself, and I was back in a major flare by late May of 2002. I waited a while before telling my gastroenterologist (a mistake) and went back on the SCD in a very strict way. In June I started using corticosteroid enemas as a way of avoiding oral steroids, and I responded well until October.

Unfortunately, the flare reached full-blown proportions in October, and the diet didn't seem to be helping. I told my gastroenterologist, and I was back to 60 mg of prednisone. Predictably, my eyesight worsened, and, after I tested my blood sugar levels, I found that I was diabetic again. Back to my GP, back to the endocrinologist, and back to the insulin. We also had the recurrent discussion about a possible colectomy, which I continued to resist. I didn't like the idea of having to wear a bag for the rest of my life to remove my body's wastes. I would do it if I absolutely had to, but this wasn't the sort of "cure" I was looking for.

Eventually, with the aid of nightly prednisone enemas, the flare subsided. This time I tried to stay on the diet rigorously. I had learned my lesson and wasn't about to take any more chances. A May 2004 colonoscopy revealed no evidence of active colitis, and I was feeling better than I had in years. I became a bit less rigorous about my diet.

Of course I flared again. I went back to strict adherence to the diet and started using the steroid enemas again. I also continued to take 100 mg of 6mp daily, and this flare resolved with the steroid enemas. A September 2005 colonoscopy showed the disease in remission.

In February of 2006, I started flaring again after beginning an aggressive exercise program. Once more I began the enemas and my gastroenterologist suggested I look into probiotics. I did, but the probiotics didn't seem to help at all. A colonoscopy in March of 2006 revealed active colitis. My gastroenterologist was not willing to put me on prednisone again—the side effects were simply too damaging for me. He was also concerned about my continuing use of steroid enemas. We discussed Remicade, which was new on the market and, at that time, was approved only for Crohn's Disease, not ulcerative colitis. This drug treatment was incredibly expensive and had its own set of potentially devastating side effects. He shook his head a number of times, paused for quite a while and then reminded me that nicotine had been useful for me in the past. I had told Ellen about my experience with nicotine, and she had already been encouraging me to explore smoking a pipe to see if that would work to keep the flares under control. I was still opposed to the idea of using tobacco because of the potential side effects and because of the social stigma surrounding smoking, but the doctor pointed out that I was in my mid-50s now, and that the potential side effects of smoking would probably do less damage than the drugs I was taking. I told him I'd think about it.

I started doing the research. My doctor had given me some medical studies in the mid-90s that seemed to show a link between nicotine and remission of ulcerative colitis. I started using a transdermal nicotine patch but didn't see much improvement, so I researched various delivery systems and discovered that pipe smokers actually seemed to live longer than non-smokers. More research helped me find sources of chemical-free, pesticide-free, organic tobacco. I knew that there was also research pointing to the chemicals in commercially-produced cigarettes as potent carcinogens. Finally, in April of 2006, I decided to buy a pipe, some chemical-free tobacco, and give it a try.

Within three days my flare started subsiding and within a week I was completely symptom-free. I continued to take 100 mg of 6mp daily, and an October 2006 blood test revealed that (as in some earlier tests) my white blood count was low. Then a November, 2006 visit showed me to be in complete remission. In September of 2007 I stopped taking the 6mp, even though my gastroenterologist wasn't happy about this. I am now off of all medications except nicotine. By the time I stopped the 6mp, Ellen had suffered a number of miscarriages, which we suspect were due to the 6mp. I was also worried about the effects of this drug on my system after so many years of being on the 6mp.

I have not had a flare since I started smoking. I still eat a low carbohydrate diet although I've included a number of foods that aren't allowed on the rigorous SCD and even occasionally treat myself to something such as ice cream, although I'm rabid about making sure that it doesn't contain carrageenan. I no longer take ANY prescription medications and not much more than an occasional antihistamine for allergies. I continue to have yearly colonoscopies (May 2007, August 2008, October 2009, and August 2011) and, after my 2009 colonoscopy, my doctor said that if he hadn't diagnosed me himself and followed my struggles for years, he would never have believed that I had been diagnosed with ulcerative colitis. My colon was completely healthy. A colonoscopy in 2011 also revealed a completely health colon. I never eat brown rice or anything that contains carrageenan, and I avoid salad and beans. When at home I cook my vegetables thoroughly, but I often eat al dente vegetables to no ill effect when out. I eat a high-fat, high-protein, low-carbohydrate diet and avoid processed foods. I smoke a pipe filled with organic tobacco. That's it.

    I can't recommend that anyone else use nicotine. For me that was a difficult, but effective, personal choice made under the supervision of my physician. Perhaps more important than this decision is the care with which I avoid carrageenan, fiber, brown rice, and other foods that have caused problems for me in the past. I try not to eat gluten as a general rule. As I've tried to make clear, smoking a pipe, along with diet, avoiding specific additives, and learning to manage stress have worked for me. I discovered this solution with the guidance of my gastroenterologist, and under no circumstances should you work in opposition to your physician or without doctor supervision and consent. One thing that I do believe is important is to become an active agent in the healing process and to be willing to look at this disease from an environmental perspective that includes diet and the full landscape of your life. Each of us should make our own decisions based on our health, goals, and beliefs, and what works for us. Be active in your work with your physicians and make sure your voice is not only heard, but valued.

    I've learned a lot on this path, and some of it is never addressed in the multitude of books available on IBD and IBS and auto-immune diseases in general. I'm sharing what's worked for me in the hope that I might help some readers develop a new, integrated way of envisioning and living with IBD and other auto-immune illnesses. It's important that we make peace with our lives and live them to the fullest, and to do that we must accept what we're dealing with while continuing to explore ways to bring the disease under control and perhaps even eliminate it.

May you become an active participant in your own health and well-being. I wish you the best.

Chapter 2
Defining Inflammatory Bowel Disease: Ulcerative Colitis and Crohn's Disease

It is difficult to get a man to understand something when his salary depends upon his not understanding it.
   Upton Sinclair. *I, Candidate for Governor: And How I Got Licked* (1935).

The best and most current book I've found on Inflammatory Bowel Disease was published in 2010 by the American Gastroenterological Association (AGA): *IBD Self-Management: The AGA Guide to Crohn's Disease and Ulcerative Colitis* by Sunanda V. Kane. This book provides the most up-to-date information on how IBD is currently defined, what is known about its causes, treatments and medications for IBD, potential extra-intestinal manifestations of IBD, surgery, diet, and lifestyle. Other useful books for the standard view of these diseases are *100 Questions and Answers About Crohn's Disease and Ulcerative Colitis* (2nd edition) by Andrew S. Warner and Amy E. Barton and *The First Year: Crohn's Disease and Ulcerative Colitis* (2nd edition) by Jill Sklar.

As I've noted repeatedly, it is crucial for all IBD patients to be in close contact with their physicians and to have as much knowledge of the disease as possible. Traditional medical approaches work very well for many people with these diseases and for those people these are probably the best books available. All three of these books stress the importance of patients taking control of the disease and their lives and give straightforward commonsense advice about living with the illness. Among the books listed above, Kane's book has the best advice about diet and living with inflammatory bowel disease.

As traditionally defined, inflammatory bowel disease (IBD) is a chronic, lifelong inflammation of the lining of the digestive system. In Crohn's disease this may be limited to either the small intestine or the large intestine or it may be present throughout the digestive tract, even the mouth. Crohn's is typically labeled according to its location and character. Someone like me, however, whose disease is limited to inflammation in the large intestine would be diagnosed as having ulcerative colitis (Kane 34). Of course, this diagnosis may change. I was originally diagnosed as having proctitis because the inflammation was limited to the lower part of the large intestine. Then it shifted to left-sided ulcerative colitis because it was present in the descending part of the large intestine. Then it became pancolitis because the entire large intestine was inflamed and ulcerated.

It's important to know what you have, but I suggest you consult your physician and books written by medical experts for this information. All I'm providing is a sort of orientation or map of this labyrinthine landscape.

Most people who are diagnosed with IBD are between the ages of 15 and 35 or 50 and 55, although very young children have also been diagnosed with IBD as have people who fall outside the age ranges specified above—I was about 40 when I was diagnosed, although I think I actually had my first episode at age of 22 or 23. The number of Americans with IBD is more than one million, with about half of them having Crohn's and half of them having ulcerative colitis. Kane points out that each year about 10 people per 100,000 are diagnosed with Ulcerative Colitis and about 16 people per one hundred thousand are diagnosed with Crohn's. Warner and Barto note that before 1960 ulcerative colitis was the most common form of IBD, but now Crohn's occurs about equally with ulcerative colitis (location 450 on Kindle) and that approximately 75 to 150 people per 100,000 people have inflammatory bowel disease. Kane also notes that IBD strikes men and women in equal numbers and that even though traditionally this has been a disease that has been associated with people of European descent and especially people of Jewish heritage, that seems to be changing as more and more African-Americans and Latinos are being diagnosed with the disease (Kane 6). Knowing which kind of IBD you have is important. The small and large intestines perform very different functions and react differently to diet and medical treatments. Since the symptoms of both Crohn's and ulcerative colitis are similar, you will need to have a doctor tell you which type of inflammatory bowel disease you have.

The origins of this disease are still unclear, but research is being carried on in attempts to understand why people get Inflammatory Bowel Disease. The main areas of research explore whether there is a genetic component, the immune system of the body, and potential environmental causes.

Genetics may play a role in the disease, although even this is uncertain. Scientists are studying certain genes to see whether or not these genes (especially if they are defective) play a role in the etiology of the disease. No definitive evidence has been found for this, and IBD always involves factors other than genetics.

IBD is an autoimmune disease and so, by definition, the immune system is involved. Again it's unclear why this happens, but the immune system seems to overreact to a perceived danger and then attacks the body rather than foreign invaders, such as bacteria, and perhaps even gluten, that pose a threat to the body. This is why immunosuppressants such as 6 mercaptopurine are sometimes effective as treatment for IBD.

Sklar and Kane note that environmental issues also play a role in IBD. Environmental factors could involve everything from smoking (bad for Crohn's but apparently good for ulcerative colitis), to food allergies, to bacteria and an upset of the bacteria in the gut (often linked to taking antibiotics), to a reaction to NSAIDs. Rarely will a physician mention stress as a cause of IBD, but just about every person who suffers from this disease knows that stress can trigger a flare, if not the disease itself. I think one of the reasons doctors say stress doesn't play a significant role in the disease is an attempt to spare patients from blaming themselves for having developed the disease. This is certainly laudable, but it's still good to try to keep the stress in your life to a minimum. I think it's useful to keep a stress journal along with your food journal to find out what role stress plays in your experience with this disease. One of the biggest causes of stress is our thinking. Are your thoughts often negative? Do your thoughts recycle unhappy experiences from the past? It might be time to get off that hamster wheel of negativity.

Standard treatments

The medical establishment offers a number of approaches to treating Inflammatory Bowel Disease. Some of these treatments have been in use for a number of years while others are relatively new. Individuals react differently to these medications and what works for one person may not work for another. Some people will experience side effects that prevent them from following standard treatments, and others will be fine with them. Keep a close eye on how your symptoms respond and make sure to do any blood tests that your gastroenterologist tells you are necessary. Even if you go into a long remission, keep in mind that inflammatory bowel diseases are not seen as curable—only treatable.

The typical first treatment will probably be with an aminosalicylate drug. These are anti-inflammatories and although they share similarities with aspirin, ibuprofen, and NSAIDS, they work in a different way and address the lining of the intestines. These drugs don't have any impact on the immune system. The most common of these are sulfasalazine, mesalamine, balsalazide, and olsalazine (Kane, 63, Sklar 105-108). The first thing my doctor tried with me was sulfasalazine, and it helped my symptoms, but the side effects were significant enough that he quickly took me off this drug. The second treatment was mesalamine, but this also had significant side effects for me. Finally, he tried mesalamine enemas (Rowasa), but these didn't help me. Many people seem to tolerate these drugs well, but I didn't. These drugs seem to be more effective with ulcerative colitis than with Crohn's disease.

Antibiotics are sometimes used—especially if your gastroenterologist suspects that a bacterium called *clostridium difficile (C. difficile)* is a contributing factor to the disease. The most common antibiotics used in treating IBD are metronidazole (Flagyl) and ciprofloxacin. Flagyl can have significant side effects. My doctor tried three or four different courses of Flagyl on me while I was in different flares, but I never saw any improvement from this treatment. Perhaps that means I didn't have a C. difficile overgrowth.

If you don't respond to the above treatments or if your symptoms are severe, the next step is probably going to be oral steroids. These are inexpensive and usually work pretty quickly. The most common of these is prednisone. High doses of prednisone always worked to bring my symptoms under control. Unfortunately, the side effects for me were so bad that I had to find an alternative treatment. I actually came to enjoy some of the effects of prednisone such as the immense amount of energy and, for me at least, a sense of well-being. However, I also had truly devastating side effects such as steroid-induced diabetes, eventually making this drug unusable for me. Long-term steroid use is associated with a range of frightening side effects. For IBD sufferers steroids are normally administered at a high initial dose, followed by a long period of decreasing the dosage each week. This is known as a "taper" or as "tapering off." The first time I tried prednisone we started with an initial dose of 40 mg per day, but when that was ineffective, we moved to 60 mg per day, and that's what all of my later rounds of prednisone would start with. I would generally taper off the drug by decreasing the dosage 2.5 mg per week. Steroids may also be administered intravenously if you have the misfortune to be hospitalized. Kane points out that the side effects of short-term steroid use could include, "weight gain, mood swings, acne, hair loss, problems with blood flow to the larger joints, an increased risk for infections, increased appetite and energy level and higher levels of blood glucose" as well as insomnia. These drugs can also create a powerful sense of well-being or a bad depression (Kane 67, Warner and Barto locations 1013-1077). Warner and Barto point out that prednisone has many short-term side effects including insomnia, acne, fluid retention, appetite increase and weight gain (Warner and Barton, location 1044). Kane says that long-term effects can include "thinning of the skin, easy bruising, osteoporosis, steroid-induced diabetes, hypertension, and cataracts" (67). It's easy to see why I initially resisted using prednisone, and why I later had to stop using it—permanently. It's also easy to see how some of the "positive" side effects can seduce its users into agreeing to frequent rounds of therapy with the drug.

Steroids are sometimes administered as an enema. When I used prednisone in this way, I had far fewer side effects. This delivery system for steroids only works on the lower bowel. Steroids are sometimes given as Entocort EC (budesonide) rather than prednisone (Kane, 68-9, Warner and Barto 1095). This steroid doesn't have the typical side effects and is sometimes effective with Crohn's disease. I tried this, but it didn't help my symptoms at all.

Another type of drug therapy involves drugs that modulate the immune system, immunomodulators. The two most common for inflammatory bowel disease are 6-mercaptopurine (6mp) and azathioprine. I took 6mp for about ten years, and it was helpful to me although it didn't keep me free from flares. It's important to remember that this drug has been linked with a potentially increased chance of developing lymphoma. When a flare did occur while I was on 6mp, I always had to use prednisone to bring it under control. I did have fewer flares while taking 6mp and did not discontinue it until well after I had started using nicotine as an alternative and effective treatment. My gastroenterologist was not pleased with me for going off of this drug, but I'm glad I did because of the potential side effects. Short term side effects could include fever, rash, joint pains, and inflammation of the pancreas (Kane 70, Warner and Barto, 1110-1140). Long term side effects can be a decreased white blood cell count while on 6mp. I had to have monthly blood draws and tests to check my white blood cell count. These drugs can also cause liver damage and have been associated with lymphoma. Another possibility, especially for men, is impact on the reproductive system. I had three healthy children in my twenties. After Ellen and I married and while I was on 6mp, we had three official miscarriages, and our OB-GYN thought the 6mp was probably responsible for these. Clearly immunomodulators have a serious downside. Methotrexate and Cyclosporin are also immunomodulators that are sometimes used for IBD. These are usually given by injection or intravenously rather than orally like 6mp.

  The last kind of treatment is known as biologics, which are used for cases of IBD that aren't responding to any of the treatments listed above. Kane says that biologic therapy has been "revolutionary," and Warner and Barto describe them as "the newest and most exciting medications used to treat IBD" (Kane 72, Warner and Barto, 1170). Rather than being chemicals, these are a special kind of protein that are cultivated in a laboratory and administered intravenously. Biologics must be administered repeatedly, typically once a month and involve about an hour-long session while the drug is administered. Remicade is used primarily for Crohn's Disease although it has also been used successfully for ulcerative colitis. This biologic is 75 percent human and 25 percent mouse protein. I have never used these although I explored Remicade and didn't feel too good about putting mouse proteins in my body. I also haven't used either of the other two biologics that are administered for IBD: Adalimumab (Humira) or Cimzia. These last two are 100 percent human protein and are administered by injection. These biologics have been used more extensively in treating Crohn's disease than in ulcerative colitis.

One of the biggest drawbacks to these biologics is their cost, about 5000 dollars a treatment or 60,000 dollars a year. I hope you have good insurance. The potential side effects also need to be considered. These can range from allergic reactions such as hives or shortness of breath to bad joint pain and swelling (Kane 74). All of the biologics are also associated with an increased risk of infections. Finally, like the immunomodulators, these are associated with an increased risk of lymphoma. A new biologic called Natalizumab (Tysabri) is, according to Kane, also available. It was approved as a treatment for multiple sclerosis but has also proven effective for Crohn's disease. Kane notes, however, "Tysabri has one side effect that unfortunately makes it somewhat unpopular: its association with a very serious infection that affects the brain" (76). As Kane points out, "Every treatment decision is a balancing act between benefit and risk, but then, most decisions are" (77).

Warner and Barto note that patients who are in remission and stay on their medications "have an 80 to 90% chance of staying in remission, whereas those who stop taking medication have an 80 to 90% chance of having an exacerbation [flare] within a year" (1343). My experience was that I could expect two or three flares a year even if I stayed on medication. By the way, you're expected to stay on these medications for the rest of your life.

Gastroenterologists hold that there is no cure for Crohn's disease, but they do offer the possibility of a cure for ulcerative colitis. The cure is removal of the colon—a colectomy. This can become necessary when ulcerative colitis is flaring and threatening the life of the sufferer, but some people choose to have the colon removed as a way of relieving the terrible symptoms that accompany the disease. This "cure" necessitates a colostomy (wearing a bag outside the body to collect the feces that are draining from the body) for the rest of the patient's life.

And you're still wondering why I was willing to see if nicotine was effective for me?

You should avoid some drugs if you have IBD. These include common drugs such as aspirin and ibuprofen (both of which caused flares for me) and all non-steroidal anti-inflammatory drugs (NSAIDS). All of these are frequently prescribed, but they all irritate the digestive system and can lead to flares.

The Crohn's & Colitis Foundation of America (CCFA) was founded in 1967 and is the group most physicians recommend a newly-diagnosed sufferer turn to. If you're interested in standard allopathic treatments or in knowing what the latest findings are from the traditional scientific and medical communities, this is a useful source and has a good website at ccfa.org. Don't expect anything other than standard information from this organization and keep in mind that it employs many people whose jobs are dependent on maintaining the status quo. De Lamar Gibbons reports that when he called the CCFA offices to discuss his theory about the dangers of fructose, he received the following response: "I was curtly informed that they were not interested in any cures and asked to please not bother them anymore. It took a little while to realize why they were so arrogant and not interested in a cure—the status quo would change and some would lose their jobs and retirement plans" (134-35). Gibbons reports a similar experience when he spoke to a gastroenterologist at the hospital where he worked about the successes he had been having treating inflammatory bowel disease and asked if the doctor had some patients who might benefit from the treatment. The reply was:

"Listen, De," he said. "I have a wife and kids to feed. These patients come in faithfully each week. They pay for my services. If you have a cure—I don't want to hear about it." He then walked off. (Beware, this could be your doctor!)

This attitude is not uncommon in medicine. Consider the consequences of the discovery of a shot or pill that would cure colitis. Established practices and treatments would change radically. Internists and gastroenterologists would lose their money-making routines and have to learn new methods (134).

My cynicism hasn't quite reached the level of Gibbons', but as a physician he has had more direct experience with the ideology of contemporary medicine than I do. Perhaps the Upton Sinclair quote at the head of this chapter deserves some thought.

Chapter 3
Diet: Standard Approaches and Some Alternatives

We're all familiar with the term "political correctness," but I'd like to suggest that we also think in terms of dietary correctness as an analogous concept. The nutritionists who have dominated our public discussion of diet have created a form of dietary correctness. This dietary correctness makes it almost impossible to speak in a positive way about some foods, such as animal fats, foods that sustained our ancestors for hundreds of thousands of years. This same dietary correctness makes it difficult to speak in a negative way about other foods such as grains, legumes, and soybeans.

Dietary recommendations by the traditional approach to medicine can be problematic although more and more gastroenterologists seem to be willing to at least consider that food might have something to do with the development and progress of inflammatory bowel disease. Diet is certainly something that every IBD sufferer is aware of and probably comes close to obsessing over since intuitively and through observation we've all learned that some foods seem to trigger flares. The conundrum is finding a diet that will provide good nutrition without bothering the gut. Unfortunately almost all of the books that deal with inflammatory bowel disease, and especially those that promise self-healing, follow the recommendations of the nutritionism establishment, and this is particularly true for those that are on the earthier side of things—

those diets that show up in birkenstocks and woolen socks. Typically these recommend such extremes as a vegan diet based primarily on raw foods and lots of fiber or lots of healing teas and supplements.

The statement "Food does not cause inflammatory bowel disease" (ibdcrohns.about.com/od/dietandnutrition/f/dieted.htm retrieved May 28, 2011) appears over and over and over again in the standard approaches to diet and inflammatory bowel disease. It's possible that there is no one specific food that causes IBD, but once more the narrow focus of current medical and scientific practice blinds researchers and physicians to the landscape of our current diet practices—a landscape that is saturated with processed foods, inedible fiber, and foods refined to the point that the only nutrition in them comes from a variety of additives. Our bodies haven't had the time to adapt to a diet of this nature—hence the "diseases of civilization" hypothesis.

Jill Sklar points out that much of this due to the training (or lack of training) provided by medical schools. Medical schools do not teach doctors about diet and nutrition—what minuscule portion of med school training is provided is based on the recommendations of the experts from the village of nutritionism:

> In textbooks on GI diseases, huge portions are dedicated to the pathological implications of the disease, the effects of the various medications, and the spectacular array of surgical options, but one thin chapter is devoted to diet. IBD textbooks are no different. Within the one chapter on diet, much information will be given on enteral feeding, the proper mixture and additives to TPN, and the effects of short bowel syndrome, but nothing is offered on giving nutrition advice of suggestions to patients who fall short of those dire circumstances (157).

Perhaps that's a blessing—at least it's a tiny bit less indoctrination in the standard western diet.

The website of the Crohn's Colitis Foundation provides information about diet and inflammatory bowel disease at www.ccfa.org/info/diet but takes the standard institutionalized medical approach:

> Patients often believe that their disease is caused by, and can be cured by diet. Unfortunately, that seems to be too simplistic an approach, which is not supported by clinical and scientific data. Diet can certainly affect symptoms of these diseases, and may play some role in the underlying inflammatory process, but it appears not to be the major factor in the inflammatory process (retrieved May 28, 2011).

This website (the leading website devoted to supporting current approaches to IBD) claims with no qualification that specific foods do not worsen the inflammation of IBD and that the key point is to eat a healthy and balanced diet (based on the recommendations of nutritionism).

> A balanced diet should contain a variety of foods from all food groups. Meat, fish, poultry, and dairy products, if tolerated are sources of protein; bread, cereal starches, fruits, and vegetables are sources of carbohydrate; margarine and oils are sources of fat. (retrieved May 28, 2011).

This website even manages to find a place for 'fast' or 'junk' food" in the IBD diet. And that's about it from this leading source of information about inflammatory bowel disease. CCFA does note that "Eating to help the gut heal itself is one of the new concepts in IBD treatment. . . " and then proceeds to recommend such foods as white bread, white rice, Gatorade, Crystal Light, fruit juices, cereals, and refined pastas (May 28, 2011). At least this website recommends avoiding high-fiber foods and prunes.

In *IBD Self-Management*, Sunanda V. Kane also accepts the recommendations of nutritionism and notes that, "Most nutrition experts say that a healthy, well-balanced diet has between half and three-quarters of its foods as carbohydrates . . ." (145-6). She does point out that even though the media generally present fat as bad, fats are important to a good diet which should include 20 to 35 percent of the calories from fat. Her recommendation follows the standard recommendation to avoid saturated fats and try to use polyunsaturated fats.

Kane further notes that when IBD is active, people need to modify their diets and should especially avoid "trigger" foods. She also recommends avoiding fiber during a flare although states that "once you are healed, fiber is part of a healthy diet" (149). She also recommends keeping a food diary to help know how you respond to particular foods and to watch for trends in that diary.

Kane devotes several pages to fiber and notes that fiber in the large intestine produces both water and gas as well as mentioning that harsher fibers can scrape the wall of the large intestine. She then says

> Fiber is good for you and, especially for its role as the producer of SCFAs [short chain fatty acids], a necessary component of a healthy diet. It is one of those foods that your body needs for long-term gut health but, at certain times, you must avoid in order to give your inflamed gut a rest. As you can see, it pays to be fiber 'savvy'! (153).

This is a good example of how the standard approach can sometimes be problematic. I've explored fiber in a separate chapter, but very little research actually supports fiber as necessary for human digestion, and personal experience will quickly show that fiber is something best avoided—no matter what the standard recommendation claim. Gary Taubes and Barry Groves both provide detailed analyses of fiber and how in the last fifty years it has come to be considered an important part of a healthy diet. The story of fiber is a story of propaganda and unfounded claims that benefits practically no one but industrial food producers.

Other issues that are often addressed by standard recommendations are the possibility of being lactose intolerant (lactose is a sugar). The recommendation is to avoid all milk products including cheese and yogurt. Be aware that it's possible to destroy the lactose in yogurt by fermenting the yogurt for 24 hours. Most hard cheese have no lactose since the lactose is destroyed by the cheese making process. Cheese and yogurt are staples in my diet and don't cause me any problems.

Kane also repeats some of the standard advice about diet not really being that important, especially for ulcerative colitis: "it is unlikely that what you eat will contribute significantly to controlling the actual inflammatory process that is occurring" (160). Technically this may be true in the midst of a flare, but diet is central to the healthy working of the body and its systems, and some foods such as sugar and gluten may make a flare worse. This is also true for some food additives such as carrageenan.

The traditional approach to diet and IBD, which finds little connection between the two, does seem to be loosening a bit. Kane, for instance, does point out that gluten can produce an autoimmune reaction which results in celiac disease or celiac sprue and notes that some people with IBD respond positively to removing gluten from the diet. The reason she gives for this, though, is that as a result of removing gluten IBD sufferers are eating more fresh foods and cooking more meals at home which is a healthier way to eat (160-61). She concludes this section by stating, "There are just so many different kinds of people who have IBD, with varied diets and sources of calories, that it seems very unlikely that we will find that a common dietary item is behind the symptoms" (161), and she's right. There probably is no single dietary item behind IBD, but our diets are part of an overall food ecology, and the food ecology most of us are consuming today is filled with processed foods and a huge variety of additives. Here again, it's important to look at the entire dietary landscape rather than isolated bits of that terrain.

One interesting development over the last ten years is that a number of books explore diets that have been proposed as candidates for healing IBD. Kane looks at three of these including the Specific Carbohydrate Diet (SCD), the Maker's Diet, and Eating for Your Blood Type. I know very little about the second and third diets, but I did follow the Specific Carbohydrate Diet religiously for two years. I found it useful in some ways, but not so useful in others. It certainly didn't heal IBD for me although it did help mitigate symptoms—or seemed to. I was also taking 6mp at the time and continued to have flares. I still follow some of the principles of the diet such as avoiding most complex carbohydrates. Kane says that the Specific Carbohydrate Diet isn't harmful but also that it is so complex and demanding that most people will have trouble following it. That was my experience. This SCD diet demands a total commitment, and if you try to follow it strictly, you will soon find that your life revolves around food and its preparation. I'm particularly bothered by its rigidity and the doctrinaire views with which some people approach it. I was on a listserv for the diet for years, and it seemed to provide some help to many people, but rare indeed were those who claimed to have been "healed" by the diet. Almost everyone was still struggling with the flares yet steadfast in the belief that if they just followed the rules closely enough healing would eventually come.

The Maker's Diet is a combination of a restrictive diet and guidelines from the Bible. The author says it is grounded in a "Biblically-correct lifestyle." On his website Jordan Rubin argues that the health crisis facing modern industrialized nations is primarily due to diet and argues, "Humanity's design has not changed, and neither has its nutrition requirements. Historical human nutrition and contemporary scientific studies indicate a way of nourishing the body that will attain and maintain overall health in the way it was designed" (http://www.makers-diet.net).

Unfortunately, this is another online site that wants to sell supplements to you. I find it difficult to trust in the claims made by groups with products to sell me.

Several books are now available which claim to put IBD sufferers on the road to self-healing, and diet is often central to these books. Another thing that is central to some of them are the supplements that the authors want to sell you to heal your IBD. Even though these books are often prefaced with glowing testimonials from people who have been "healed" by following the advice of the authors, I would approach these with great caution. Adding a group of expensive supplements is really just filling your gut with another kind of chemical which enriches the seller. I don't trust this approach, and it is an affront to the concept of an ecological approach to the body. To me it resembles applying synthetic pesticides, herbicides, and fertilizers to a lawn to produce a lush patch of green that's utterly artificial.

David Dahlman is a chiropractor who has written a book called *Why Doesn't My Doctor Know This? Conquering Irritable Bowel Syndrome, Inflammatory Bowel Disease, Crohn's Disease and Colitis*. Be warned: inflammatory bowel disease is given a passing glance, but Dahlman's focus is on irritable bowel syndrome—a completely different animal from inflammatory bowel disease. Unsurprisingly Dahlman attacks traditional medicine and the training physicians receive. Dahlman also wants to sell you supplements. He does make good observations about the link between traditional allopathic practitioners and the pharmaceutical companies—just before fifteen pages devoted to the supplements he recommends and will sell to you. Dahlman does, however, point out that diet must play a role in gastrointestinal diseases:

> I can't count the number of times patients have told me that their doctor or gastroenterologist said to them—with a straight face—that diet is playing no role in their IBS, Crohn's disease, or colitis symptoms. Here are specialists in the gastrointestinal system, the part of the body that processes food, who, when presented with a patient complaining of gastrointestinal symptoms, don't believe that the food the patient is eating has any relevance to the patient's symptom profile. Unbelievable! (25).

I have to agree. Dahlman has four dietary rules (for IBS):

> Avoid all dairy products (including cheese and yogurt) although he does allow butter.

Avoid gas-causing foods including all beans and cruciferous vegetables like broccoli; he also says to avoid all soy products but not to worry about soy lecithin.

Do not drink liquids during or directly after meals.

Do not take your regular vitamin, mineral, or herbal supplements.

Dahlman's single chapter on inflammatory bowel disease is not particularly helpful. He thinks cases of IBD are probably advanced cases of IBS; he believes that IBD can be reversed and healed. His suggestions are to follow the four rules I've listed above, to take his supplements, and to eliminate gluten. That's about it for IBD, although he also suggests avoiding fructose—a suggestion that comes from a book by De Lamar Gibbons, *The Self-Help Way to Treat Colitis and Other IBS Conditions*. Gibbons also believes that IBD is simply a severe case of IBS and avoiding fructose is the cornerstone of his self-healing system.

De Lamar Gibbons is a physician with an axe to grind against physicians—some of his points bear thinking about, but the basis of his self-healing program is avoiding fructose: "Fructose intolerance has been the missing piece of the irritable bowel disease puzzle" [he considers Crohn's and ulcerative colitis to be forms of irritable bowel syndrome] (79).

The problem with diets such as these is exactly the problem of over-specialization (or over focus) that I discussed in an ecological approach to illness. Gibbons is so focused on one particular thing that he overlooks the larger landscape. This book contains some of the worst diet advice for IBD I've ever read. He recommends sucrose—refined table sugar—as a friendly food for IBD sufferers. Remember that Groves and Taubes make it clear that sugar is one of the primary culprits in the diseases of civilization hypothesis which springs from the problems with the western diet. He does recommend avoiding fiber, but recommends that one substitute white bread for whole wheat bread. Although the Specific Carbohydrate Diet says potatoes must be avoided, Gibbons believes potatoes to be one of the best foods for IBD. I have never had any problems with potatoes, but it's worth remembering that potatoes are essentially starch, and starches are converted into sugar during the digestive process.

A number of other books claim to heal inflammatory bowel disease through diet, but these should be approached with caution since they often contain highly questionable and even potentially damaging information. For example in *Self Healing Colitis & Crohn's: The Complete Wholistic Guide to Healing the Gut & Staying Well* (2009), David Klein recommends a vegan diet as a healing plan and emphasizes the importance of eating foods raw rather than cooked.

The Web has an enormous amount of information available about diet and IBD, but be careful. This information is often marked by faddism and if you read much of it at all, you'll find incredible amounts of contradictory information—one site recommends soy, another says avoid it; one site recommends a whole grain diet for the fiber, of all things; others say avoid it; one site will recommend avocado, another will avoid it. This is one of the places where it pays to be a very careful and thoughtful hunter and gatherer of information. Almost all of these websites follow current fashion or faddism in one form or another—typically they warn IBD sufferers away from animal fats (one of the things needed for healing; see Groves and Taubes). I've tried to address the biggest issues in this book, but these are things that have worked for me. IBD is an individualized disease and what works for one person won't work for another. I have tried to touch upon some of the biggest causes of problems. I've also tried to present some things that can be helpful—things few writers will touch because of the current climate of thought.

Some of the most sensible advice I've come across for making food choices are from Michael Pollan and his book *In Defense of Food*. He provides a number of recommendations for eating in a healthy way, but my personal favorites are: don't eat anything your great grandmother wouldn't recognize as food; avoid food products containing ingredients that are a) unfamiliar, b) unpronounceable, c) more than five in number, or that include d) high-fructose corn syrup; shop the peripheries of the supermarket and stay out of the middle (148-157).

Chapter 4
I Am Not a Disease

Self-definition is one of the greatest powers we have, and yet it is also one that is too often taken away from us. Sometimes we even give this power away to others. In the field of post-colonial studies writers explore the effects of colonialism on the people who were subjected to domination by others. Students of post-colonialism look at how a once-subjected people recover their voice and learn to speak in their own voices rather than through the words, values, and ideas of the colonizer. A second major theme in post-colonial studies is the question of identity and the right to determine one's own identity instead of the colonizer having the power to define you and to determine the course of your life.

We can apply this metaphor of colonization to inflammatory bowel disease—indeed to all auto-immune diseases. These diseases essentially colonize not only our bodies, our intestines, our immune system, but they also colonize our identity. One of the most important things you can do for your health is to take a stand against being defined by others—demand the right to define yourself and to speak with your own voice. Throw out the invader and do not let this alien colonize your mind or your speech or your imagination.

You are not a disease.

Far too many people blame themselves for developing inflammatory bowel disease or other auto-immune diseases which, by definition, are diseases in which the body attacks itself. One of the most important gifts of the gastroenterologists I've spoken with is their emphasis that inflammatory bowel disease is not due to a certain character type and has nothing to do with the kind of people we are. Disease is not a punishment for being a particular kind of person in spite of the all-too frequent views that put the blame for illness on the patient. Nothing in your character created this betrayal by the body. Refuse to allow yourself to be defined in this way. Instead, keep searching for ways to manage and overcome the illness you are currently experiencing.

In case we're tempted to think that only those sufferers from auto-immune disease are subject to the idea that they are their illness, take a look at the pharmaceutical industry's search for new illnesses and drugs (and therefore new markets and new "clients") through what is literally the invention of new illnesses. We've all seen the ads that appear on television between five and ten pm. The vast majority of the advertisements are for prescription medications, a long list of prescription medications. Viewers, or, as the marketers see them, potential clients and patients, are repeatedly advised to "ask their doctor." For some fascinating reading take a look at articles that describe the pharmaceutical industry's search for new drugs to sell through the creation or invention of new illnesses. These new "illnesses" feature drugs that "treat" such "disorders" as "restless leg syndrome" or Social Affective Disorder (SAD) which used to be known as being shy or introverted. Are we really going to allow the pharmaceutical industry to define a character trait such as "shyness" as a personality disorder to be treated by drugs?

Chapter 5
The Ecology of Illness: An Ecological Perspective

Something has gone dreadfully wrong in the western world. Chronic illnesses, especially auto-immune diseases, are rising rapidly. If the twentieth century went down in history as the century of cancer and chronic heart disease, the twenty-first century is on the way to becoming the century of auto-immune diseases such as inflammatory bowel disease, lupus, and multiple sclerosis. How much of this is related to the changes in diet that began in the 1970s in the western world and have been accelerating since? As Datis Kharrazian points out in *Why Do I Still Have Thyroid Symptoms When my Lab Tests are Normal*, "Hippocrates said that all disease begins in the gut . . . yet gastrointestinal (GI) dysfunctions are the most overlooked and exceedingly common disorders today, affecting about 70 million Americans . . .Since most of the immune system is situated in the digestive tract, a problematic gut leads to a problematic immune system. Because the lining of the digestive tract is an important immune barrier, poor gut health is a significant factor in triggering autoimmune diseases such as Hashimoto's as well as functional hypothyroidism" (119).

I want to suggest that we consider the importance of the ecological or environmental perspective when thinking about auto-immune diseases in general and especially about inflammatory bowel disease. The most important concept in this way of thinking is to envision a variety of systems and to realize that with any complex system, the addition or removal of any element, no matter how small, is going to reverberate with consequences—some of them intended, some of them unintended.

Think of the interacting, interdependent systems that make up the body—the digestive system, the circulatory system, the respiratory system—each of which is complex in its own right. The circulatory system, for example, is composed of a four-chambered heart, a network of veins and arteries which nourish and cleanse all of the cells and organs of the body, capillaries, red and white blood cells, and much more. All of the body's systems, including the circulatory system and the digestive system, work together to create the ecology or environment of the human body.

Most of the systems that relate to our health have undergone dramatic changes in the last fifty years. In thinking ecologically about illness, we must move beyond just looking at the integrated system of the body and include nutritionism, the medical establishment, and the food industry. All of these systems together create a complex and multidimensional ecosystem with our bodies and our health at the center of the system.

An essential part of an ecological approach is observation, paying attention. Just as we would notice changes in the landscape and how these impact the various species living in that landscape, we notice changes in the ecology of our bodies. What are we putting into our bodies? What are the daily changes that we observe as we alter things such as diet or medications? Notekeeping is crucial to this process. I recommend that you buy a small notebook that you can keep with you and use it to record exactly what you eat, the medications you take, and even a record of going to the toilet. How often? Was it bloody? Was mucus present? Did you have diarrhea? Record your observations and stay aware of how the addition or subtraction of a particular element or event may have profound impacts. This record-keeping is even more crucial when it comes to healing disease since one is dealing with a number of interlocking systems: the ecology of the gut, the ecology of the body, the ecology of diet, the ecology of the medical establishment, the ecology of media and information delivery, the ecology of nutritionism, and the anarchic ecology of the World Wide Web as a source of information.

Another element in this approach is the importance of what poets such as Gary Snyder and spiritual thinkers such as Eckhart Tolle name "presence." Presence is simply awareness, but this can be much more difficult than it sounds. Presence demands focused awareness, and for those suffering from IBD this means focused awareness of the body, its signs and messages. Listen to the body and observe its reactions. The body speaks to us, but we must be willing to listen and to do the work of translating the body's messages into a language we understand. Develop a dialogue with yourself based on a profound listening and presence. The world, including our little internal planet, speaks to us all of the time. Learning to pay attention to this dialogue, this subtle "speech," opens up important channels of communication.

Illness does not take place in an isolated setting. It is a part of a larger system and is a manifestation, a sign, that something in that system is out of balance. Emerson reminds us that if we pay attention to even the small details, we learn that nothing is in-SIGN-ificant—all things are signs that speak to those who are paying attention. Aldo Leopold speaks of restoring a damaged ecosystem as "reinhabitation," and that's exactly what each of us must do—learn to consciously reinhabit our bodies in order to restore our health. Clearly the old ways of doing things aren't working. We must be open to new approaches.

Specialization has been both a blessing and a curse for our world, creating experts who are able to bring great skill and knowledge to almost any issue facing us today. However, these same experts tend to inhabit small villages of information surrounded primarily by other people who are expert in the same area—their tribe. As a result the world of knowledge today is one of many,

many small clusters of huts dotting an enormous landscape without any roads joining these villages together. The dream of our world is a dream of integration. We need these small communities of experts, but we also need to join them together, so that they are communicating and sharing insights and information. If you think of these villages as boxes, the question becomes how to tear down the walls of the boxes. These boxes or villages represent the various disciplines and specialties that make up the landscape of knowledge, but it's crucial that we discover ways to link these isolated villages. We have to find ways to integrate the knowledge from a variety of fields. This demands that "experts" stretch beyond their comfort zones and explore other villages. Otherwise the experts find themselves essentially talking only to their inner circle, reinforcing the orthodox beliefs that prevail in that particular community. In any ecosystem diversity provides strength.

Unfortunately the villages of experts that dominate our knowledge landscape have more in common with a field of corn in Kansas, a monoculture, than an old-growth climax forest which nurtures an enormous diversity of life and, as a result, is stronger as an ecosystem. The old-growth forest doesn't need to be sprayed with herbicides, fungicides, and pesticides in order to maintain a healthy ecology. This forest is also tolerant of diversity and variety, and there's no expectation that all of the plants grow in the same way. Naturally complex ecosystems are in balance and are able to restore their own health should a part of the system get out of kilter. An old-growth intellectual ecosystem would not only tolerate but welcome a variety of ideas and approaches to any problem.

This analogy can be extended even more broadly. Just as the agribusinessman who farms corn takes a totalitarian approach of extermination to all plants except his corn, a monocultural approach to knowledge tries to weed out and destroy any ideas that conflict with or threaten the dominant ideological ecosystem by trying to shut down or exterminate those ideas. This is simply the way systems (or the "system") work. I don't know about you, but I'd much prefer to live among the splendor and richness of an old-growth forest than in the middle of a monocultured field of wheat, corn, or soybeans, genetically modified and all cultivated from the same seed engineered in a lab.

Those of us who are dealing with inflammatory bowel disease or any other autoimmune disease are currently living in a landscape of illness. We know this landscape well. It manifests itself in the body in pain, gas, bloating, fatigue, body aches, discomfort, frequent trips to the bathroom, blood, and a sense that we are out of control. It manifests itself in our nutritional landscape as we wonder about what foods we should be eating and whether those foods are helping or hurting our illness. It manifests itself in our medical landscape as we surrender control of our lives to a medical bureaucracy that attempts to "manage" our illness as though it were a faceless, nameless assortment of problems that can be "solved" if just the right combination of management techniques can be discovered and applied to the "problem." It manifests itself in the landscape of the drugs that we're putting into our bodies, generating enormous profits for the pharmaceutical companies who are much more interested in treating our symptoms for as long as we live than in finding a cure that would resolve the illness and thus remove the need for profitable drugs. It manifests itself in the industrial landscape of the processed food industry that dominates food production in the western world and whose primary goal is to produce food as cheaply as possible (even if that means selling us what is literally industrial waste) and to sell that "food" at the highest profit margin.

All of these systems have joined to produce an unholy and unhealthy alliance that has you at the center. You are a "consumer" contributing to their bottom line. Meanwhile your "bottom" line is fundamentally compromised.

Seeing the self as an ecological system involves more than just the body and how we think of it. This vision must also include our mind, and that means the imaginative mind and the rational mind as well as our spirit. By spirit I don't mean a particular religious point of view but simply the recognition that we are spiritual beings as well as physical beings, and this aspect of our well-being must be part of our ecological vision. All of these elements make up who we are and should be addressed as seriously as the physical body. We are more than bags of skin filled with organs and fluids, even though that's how many of us have found ourselves treated and may even be the way we've come to think of ourselves.

If you take nothing else from this book, please take this: the control of information is the control of power. Totalitarianism works through the control of information. This is the method used by all totalitarian systems whether it's an institution (insert your own favorite repressive institution here) or a dictatorial regime such as those of Germany under the Nazis or North Korea today. We certainly don't live under political or religious dictatorships, but we do inhabit a world in which information about such topics as nutrition and health is controlled by a new priesthood which maintains its power by keeping us confused and uninformed. I don't think these people are usually doing this intentionally, but they do have a vested interest in maintaining a position of power in which they have the "truth" and the rest of us don't. Unfortunately, much of the information they pass on as though it were religious dogma is bad information, based on out-moded or bad science, a faulty system which is making us increasingly obese and increasingly unhealthy.

One of the most important books in the history and philosophy of science in the last fifty years is *The Structure of Scientific Revolutions* by Thomas S. Kuhn (1962). In this groundbreaking and seminal work, Kuhn attempts to understand how science works as well as how scientific knowledge changes over time and, sometimes, moves forward. One of the fundamental truths Kuhn points out is that no "scientific group could practice its trade without some set of received beliefs" (4). Received beliefs in science are analogous to the same concept in religion. These are the beliefs that practitioners accept as "truth," beliefs that guide the practitioners of both science and religious practice. These accepted "truths" provide the concept of orthodoxy—a concept as important in science as in religion. Kuhn explores how the received beliefs of science both determine the way scientists ply their trade and how shifts, or revolutions, take place in the way scientists conceive of science or even what topics constitute the proper subjects of scientific study. For instance, Newton's vision of a scientific universe made up of eternal and unchanging laws that governed the properties of all physical things dominated the scientific world for centuries until it was replaced with the evolutionary model proposed by Darwin. Both of these models are still available to scientists, and the evolutionary model is particularly relevant today. However, another revolution in the received beliefs of science occurred with the twentieth century shift toward quantum mechanics. The received beliefs or orthodoxy of any scientific community determine how that community practices science. Kuhn points out that these beliefs are the foundation of a scientist's education, and that the "rigorous and rigid" education scientists go through guarantees that the received beliefs have a powerful hold on the future scientist's mind and work to keep the scientist from questioning those beliefs (5).

What Kuhn calls "normal science" (orthodoxy) is built around the belief that the scientific community knows what the basic world is like. Scientists work hard to defend beliefs. For instance, Newton's vision of the universe was a mechanistic one. The universe was a giant machine set in motion by God, functional like the wheels and cogs in a giant clock that operated according to unchanging and eternal laws. The revolution precipitated by Darwin replaced that static and mechanical vision with a dynamic, evolutionary model that could be better described as a bush—a bush with a multitude of branches that was always in the process of growth. Kuhn further points out that, "normal science often suppresses fundamental novelties because they are necessarily subversive of its basic commitments" (5). In other words, just as in the case of religious believers, scientists are resistant to changes in their basic belief system about how the world and the universe work, and almost all scientific research is "a strenuous and devoted attempt to force nature into the conceptual boxes supplied by professional education" (5).

Two crucial concepts for Kuhn's theory are *normal science* and *paradigms*. Kuhn defines "normal science" as "research firmly based upon one or more past scientific achievements, achievements that some particular scientific community acknowledges for a time as supplying the foundation for its further practice" (10). Normal science is science that develops, extends, and strengthens the orthodox beliefs of its practitioners. This set of beliefs is what Kuhn refers to as a paradigm. Think of a paradigm as a structure or a lens through which scientists view the world, the frame through which they see. By its very nature this lens has distortions and can be focused on only part of what the scientist is investigating at any one time. Occasionally, and usually after much intellectual struggle and debate, a scientific paradigm (or box of orthodox beliefs) will undergo a shift. This shift creates a fundamental change in the way scientists conceive of the universe and its underlying principles. These paradigm shifts are what Kuhn refers to as scientific revolutions.

An example of a paradigm shift took place during the early Renaissance when the Copernican vision of the universe, which placed the sun at the center of our solar system, replaced the older Ptolemaic vision, which located the earth at the center of the universe. Even though today almost everyone accepts a vision of our solar system as one composed of planets that circle the sun as well as a vision of the universe as an unfathomably complex system of galaxies of billions of stars, this was a revolutionary idea when Copernicus proposed it—an idea that ended up with Galileo being excommunicated and placed under house arrest by the Catholic Church for his refusal to renounce this belief since it conflicted with the orthodox religious and scientific beliefs of his time. It ultimately led to Galileo's death and put a halt, for a time, to other scientists who might have felt inclined to express the same, more "modern" scientific viewpoint. A current example of what happens when a paradigm shift takes place is the continuing conflict over evolution, an idea which still sends shockwaves through American culture even though it is accepted by the world-wide scientific community. For Kuhn a scientific revolution is "the tradition-shattering complements to the tradition-bound activity of normal science" (6). New scientific theories force scientists to rebuild their earlier assumptions and evaluations of "facts" to transform the landscape of science and how it is practiced.

Kuhn's model makes it clear that science is an inherently conservative way of knowing the world and that most scientific research is dedicated to reinforcing the paradigm that currently rules any particular scientific era. The problem with this is that it becomes extraordinarily difficult for anyone, but especially for scientists, to effect a change in a particular paradigm or scientific way of defining the world. The existing paradigm impacts literally everything about the way science is practiced, including the kinds of questions that are asked and the kinds of answers that are therefore found. Try to keep these ideas of normal science (orthodoxy) and paradigms (ways of seeing) in mind when thinking about the information given to our society about what constitutes a "healthy" diet. Also try to remember this when thinking about the way medicine is practiced and about the assumptions that underlie current approaches to disease, including specific diseases such as inflammatory bowel disease.

Each of us has a set of lenses through which we view the world, even if we aren't scientists. These lenses are shaped by the orthodox beliefs about such things as diet that are spread through instituions such as the mass media. For example, we might think about the diets adopted by people who are trying to be ethical and leave the fewest traces on the world. These diets are often based primarily on grains and are among the least healthy and least natural for the human digestive system. Unfortunately this dietary approach is associated with the environmentalist world view and many, many people who think they're doing a good thing for the world by consuming low-fat, high-fiber, carbohydrate-based diets are doing horrible things to themselves. Save the world through self-sabotage and self-destruction? This seems like neither a workable nor a moral approach.

It's difficult to find oneself struggling against orthodoxy—a set of beliefs that are accepted in the same way religious beliefs are accepted, but too often these are unexamined ideas that have come to hold a central, almost holy, place in our belief system because they have been adopted by like-minded people and have come to feel "right," and even "true." Many of the ideas in this book are blasphemous when viewed from the orthodox nutritionist perspective. Please don't just take my word for the things I present here. Do your own research, but do the research with an open mind. Don't allow your mind to shut down if an idea is uncomfortable or doesn't fit with the dogma presented by the voices that currently dominate our cultural discussion. All knowledge, including scientific knowledge, is built on a set of assumptions that are often unexamined and are always subject to change. Just think of how often a piece of information about diet and health is presented and then overturned with the opposite information now presented as true. Remember eggs? They're bad for you. Wait, they're the ultimate food! Coffee is a good example. A few years ago, we were told it was bad for us and that we shouldn't drink more than a cup a day, if that. Then we were told that drinking coffee apparently protects against Alzheimer's. Recently we were told that drinking six cups of coffee a day seems to provide protection against prostate cancer. On the other hand, coffee might create problems for the heart and sinus rhythm. Confused yet?

The reversals around such things as eggs or coffee provide a pretty good window into the current state of nutritionism and medical wisdom about our diets. It also doesn't hurt to remember that most physicians didn't take even one course on nutrition and nutrition's relationship to health in medical school—that's right, not a single class! Physicians learn most of what they know about nutrition in the same way you do—through what they hear in the media or read in magazines or current books about health, and it's always good to remember that the loudest voices in our media-saturated culture are often those with the most money behind them, with the most to gain from a particular nutritional agenda. Be sure to ask who funded the latest study you just read lauding the benefits of fiber—an inedible waste product of the food processing industry that only became part of dietary dogma in the 1970s and for which no major study (which has stood up to continued scrutiny) has ever found a heath benefit.

Another thing to keep in mind is that it's possible to find information to support just about any position imaginable if you look on the Internet. One bias most of us cart with us when we encounter new information is that we readily accept ideas that confirm our view of how the world works and we reject (or we don't even notice) information that challenges our assumptions. Please don't fall into that trap. Try to keep your mind open as you evaluate information, always remembering to follow the money trail to see which company or organization funded a particular line of research.

The intersection of nutritionism, the medical establishment, public policy, and, above all, the processed food industry has created a nutritional ecology, or village, which is not providing us with information that serves our best interests. Nutritionists aren't really to blame. They've been taught to believe that a particular way of eating is the best for us, but Gary Taubes, Michael Pollan, Loren Cordain, Barry Groves, and a number of other respected writers have made it clear that the food pyramid (or "plate," in its newest incarnation) and other commonly accepted nutritional advice is based on bad science. The food industry has a clear goal—to produce "food" as cheaply as possible and to sell this manufactured product at the highest possible prices. These companies produce "food" from the cheapest sources available—soy, corn, wheat, rice, and waste products such as bran. Too many of us are filling our bodies with what is literally industrial waste, and the result is that our digestive systems have become toxic and have attacked the bodies that contain them—the bodies they are designed to cleanse, not to destroy. This has been a boon for the medical establishment and especially for the pharmaceutical industry which begins its bribery and propagandizing of doctors on the first day of medical school and never stops. Just look around your physician's office or examining room. How many of the pens, notepads, clocks, calendars, and other items are nothing more than advertisement for a particular drug. An expensive drug. A drug that probably lists all sorts of frightening, and even potentially lethal, side effects in the fine print. This comment may sound cynical, but there's no profit to be found for anyone in the medical establishment from curing people. The profit comes from treating ongoing symptoms, and what could be more profitable than a chronic disease? This doesn't mean that physicians aren't truly caring people doing their best for their patients. They often are. I've been treated by some brilliant doctors whom I think of as friends and who have been willing to explore possible treatments with the ultimate goal of curing a chronic disease. Unfortunately many doctors are also the "priests" in a religion, and like any religious believer their actions are founded on faith. No one, not even the most dedicated and industrious doctor, has the time to explore all of the new information that deluges any professional today. Just as most politicians take the majority of their information from a group of self-interested lobbyists, physicians take much of their information from those who "should" know—the people who are creating, testing, and marketing new drugs.

  Another major issue with medicine as it is currently practiced is also one of its greatest strengths—specialization. Specialization definitely has its place and many lives are saved as a result of having practitioners who are knowledgeable about a specific system or organ; however, it's possible today for someone who has a chronic disease to find themselves seeing a number of different specialists who aren't always in close communication. Perhaps you are seeing your general practitioner, a gastroenterologist, and an endocrinologist. If you have other health issues you might also be consulting a neurologist, a cardiologist, a nephrologist, or even a dermatologist. How closely are these various physicians in contact with each other? This lack of communication can be exacerbated if you happen to live in a small town and visit your general practitioner there, then drive fifty miles to another town to see your gastroenterologist, and have to drive 250 or 350 miles to see the neurologist or endocrinologist. This is not a hypothetical scenario—I've done it. Certainly it could be argued that the general practitioner should be keeping tabs on all the medications the different practitioners prescribe for different issues, but how likely is it that the general practitioner is going to be keeping up with these specializations—especially since the general practitioners are probably already overworked and stretched to their human limits. Is anyone supervising everything? If you're unlucky, a negative drug interaction will take place, which could lead to a cascade of problems. The key person here is you. Learn from my example—I did not do a good job of keeping the specialists I was working with informed when I was prescribed a new drug and almost died on more than one occasion as a result. Had I talked to my gastroenterologist (who saw me the most often and knew the most about my health issues), I would never have started these drugs. He was horrified when he was informed because he was knowledgeable about possible side effects that could and did affect my ulcerative colitis. He also knew about some of the potential drug interactions. The problem here was not simply the way medicine is currently practiced. I had not yet become as active a participant in my own health as I should have been. I hadn't yet learned to lobby, actively and forcefully, for my own health.

Many physicians are open to alternative explorations, however, and are perfectly willing to work with patients as they explore alternatives. Do your best to find one of these physicians with an open mind who hasn't been shackled by orthodoxy and dogma.

Keep in mind the concept of an ecological vision of the world of medicine and any health challenges you might face, and remember that this is not just one ecological system but a number of interlocking systems that intertwine to form the complexity of "you." Let's live long enough and well enough to become an "old growth forest" ourselves.

Chapter 6
The Standard American Carbohydrate-Based Diet and the Diseases of Civilization

> For ninety-nine percent of human existence, people lived as foragers in small nomadic bands. Our brains are adapted to that long-vanished way of life, not to brand-new agricultural and industrial civilizations. They are not wired to cope with anonymous crowds, schooling, written language, government, police, courts, armies, modern medicine, formal social institutions, high technology, and other newcomers to the human experience.
>
> Stephen Pinker, *How the Mind Works*, p 42 (Kindle edition)

This chapter offers a brief introduction to the modern Western Diet and its relationship to the cluster of illnesses often referred to as the "diseases of civilization." I'll give an overview on some of the ways that this diet impacts and perhaps even leads to the creation of ulcerative colitis, Crohn's disease, and irritable bowel syndrome. *Good Calories, Bad Calories: Challenging the Conventional Wisdom on Diet, Weight Control, and Disease* (2007) by the award winning science writer, Gary Taubes, is the best book I've found on this topic. His book is thoroughly researched and filled with detail and information from a huge list of scientific studies as well as from a historical analysis of the problems of the Western Diet. If you read nothing else about the multitude of horrible effects of the diet most people in industrialized nations have adopted over the last 50 years, read this. It is a rigorous, rather scholarly read, but if you're going to take control of your disease, you want to be informed and need to do the work to be informed. Remember—you're no longer a passive victim in the hands of the medical, nutritional, and food industry establishments, nor of the pharmaceutical priests. Another very useful book is by the British researcher, Barry Groves. His book, titled *Trick and Treat*, addresses the problems of the Western diet and the food industry. Michael Pollan's brilliant best-seller, *In Defense of Food*, is a joy to read and also presents an indictment of the food industry, the nutritional establishment, and current medical practice. Pollan, however, recommends a diet based primarily on plant foods and some of his advice, although perhaps fine for some people suffering under the regime of the Western diet, could be problematic for those of us with Inflammatory Bowel Disease. A couple of other excellent books that focus on humans, human evolution, and diet are *The Paleo Diet: Lose Weight and Get Healthy by Eating the Food You Were Designed to Eat* by Loren Cordain (2002) and *The New Evolution Diet: What Our Paleolithic Ancestors Can Teach Us about Weight Loss, Fitness, and Aging* by Arthur De Vany (2011). All of these book are a bit easier to read than Taubes and are carefully researched and packed with important information about the diet most of us now eat.

Try to keep a few things in mind as you read this chapter and as you think about some of the information that directly conflicts with the diet we've been repeatedly told is healthy. The three things we need to be aware of are food faddism, dietary correctness (a sort of ideological orthodoxy), and propaganda.

Just as fads occur among middle school age girls and boys, fads can occur in any area of our lives such as music, fashion, or religious beliefs. Fads also occur in professions, diet, and foods.

Different foods and styles of eating come and go as fads, and these fads are responsible for much of the confusion most people feel about what constitutes a healthy diet. Was it yesterday or last week that red wine was bad for us? Today we're told that it's good for us.

What about soy? Fiber? Transfats? Polyunsaturated fats? Eggs? This faddism can contribute to real health problems. Arthur De Vany notes,

> The current debate over fat versus carbohydrate is anchored totally in the modern idea of eating. This is really an argument over fads, because virtually every modern diet is just a small variation on bad nutritional thinking (18).

Nutrition is a newer (and complex) science that still has many murky areas. Unfortunately some of the ideas that are accepted almost as items of religious belief by nutritionists today, such as the idea that animal fat is bad or that cholesterol causes heart disease, are not supported by good science. Writers like Gary Taubes, Michael Pollan, and Barry Groves present brilliant analyses of these examples of bad science. Taubes is particularly good at dissecting how some of these false and misleading ideas about nutrition entered the scientific mainstream, and he reveals the bad science behind these studies. Pollan is particularly good at exploring the origins and development of the field of nutrition and the rise of what he calls nutritionism—an approach that considers "nutrients" rather than food and is more concerned with the quantity of what we put in our bodies than the quality. Somehow, much of the discussion of nutrition rests on explanations of body weight with such misleading platitudes as "calories in, calories out," or "a calorie is a calorie." Often practically no attention is paid to the *source* of the calories—the actual things we put into our bodies to fuel them.

How did this sorry state of quasi-science in nutritionism come to exist? Remember the concept of paradigms from Thomas Kuhn and how these can come to dominate the thinking of groups such as scientists so completely that they aren't able to see beyond the limits of the paradigm that has been accepted? Sometimes these paradigms in nutrition have come to have their starring role because of a study that seemed to reveal great possibilities for a particular food such as fiber which also offered the possibility of great rewards for industrial food manufacturers. Follow-up studies disprove the supposed benefits, but the damage has already been done. Partly this is a result of a media ecology that is much better at trumpeting news of a startling new approach to improving our health than in following up with the disappointing results, better at grabbing a headline than at reading the fine print to discover who funded a study, and therefore who designed the study, and thus who is benefitting from its "conclusions."

Unfortunately this concept of paradigms also leads to orthodoxy—a commitment to the established "wisdom" that is based on faith and whose followers enforce the second thing to keep in mind: the concept of "dietary correctness." This is similar to the concept of "political correctness" that was in the news a few years ago and has the same chilling results on new ideas and the expression of ideas. If one poses a question or presents a study that challenges the faith of the orthodox, the true believers, one is probably going to encounter great resistance, even attack, from the true believers.

This is reinforced by the way science is practiced in most countries (especially the United States) today. Science and research are expensive. Most of the research projects conducted today are funded by sources such as food producers or pharmaceutical companies, businesses that have a vested interest in specific results, and if a researcher wants to continue to have funding for his or her research, in other words, to have a job, the results had better confirm what the funder is looking for. I know this sounds cynical, but a number of examples of this have come to light in recent years.

One of the most notorious recent examples involved three psychiatry professors at Harvard University Medical School who received more than a million dollars each from the drug makers Eli Lilly, Johnson & Johnson, Pfizer, GlaxoSmithKline and Bristol-

Myers Squibb. This was their "reward" for aggressively pushing the diagnosis of bipolar disorder in children. From 1994 to 2003 the diagnosis of pediatric bipolar disorder increased by forty times and with this increasing diagnosis came an enormous increase in the use of antipsychotic drugs in children (http://www.pharmalot.Com /2011/07harvard-docs-disciplined-for-conflicts-of-interest/).

Bloomberg news reported in September 2007, "The expanded use of bipolar as a pediatric diagnosis has made children the fastest-growing part of the $11.5 billion U.S. market for anti-psychotic drugs" (http://www.alternet.org/story/88333/ exposed%3A_harvard_ shrink_gets_rich_labeling_kids_bipolar).

More instances of this practice of engineered medical results have been detailed by *The New York Times*. The *Times* reported on a professor who promoted the benefits of cholesterol drugs and belittled students who asked about side effects. The author, Duff Wilson, notes that Harvard received a grade of "F" from the American Medical Student Association, a group that grades medical schools on how well they monitor and control drug industry money. Merck Pharmaceuticals has even built a corporate research center across the street from Harvard's medical research building (http://www.nytimes.com/2009/03/03/business/03medschool.html). The funders behind these studies are rarely revealed.

Pharmaceutical companies have even been known to have marketing specialists on their payroll who "invent" a disease, which is then researched by a supposedly objective scientist while the drug company develops a chemical to market for this newly-minted disease, a product which is then marketed after the disease has been "researched" and announced throughout the media sphere. The May/June 2010 issue of *Boston Review* contained a forum on the impact of the pharmaceutical industry on medical training and science which included a section on "Selling Diseases." This article notes that pharmaceutical company employees target influential medical school professors and health care professionals who are courted by the pharmaceutical company to sell not drugs, but diseases—the pharmaceutical company salespeople will then sell the actual drugs; see http://bostonreview.net/BR35.3/fugh-berman.php. We've all heard of "restless leg syndrome," but *AlterNet.org* identified eight invented diseases the pharmaceutical companies are counting on to make big profits. These included Statin Deficiency. The article notes that "Last year (2009) the FDA approved AstraZeneca's Crestor for children as young as 10 and in March it approved Crestor for 6.5 million people who have no cholesterol or problems at all!" Other invented diseases *AlterNet* identifies are circadian dysrthythmia or excessive sleepiness which can be treated by modern versions of stimulants such as Provigil, and adult autism and adult onset ADHD, both of which which require "lifelong" medication. You can read the article in its entirety at http://www.alternet.org/story/146471/8_invented_diseases_big_pharma_is_banking_on but also see *Mother Jones*, May 11, 2010, "Inventing Disease to Sell Drugs" and this website from the BBC: http://newsvote.bbc.co.uk/.

These examples from the pharmaceutical industry also hold true for nutritional claims made for many foods. The same process is repeated in industry-funded research on nutrition and diet. This is why we get "studies" finding that eating processed breakfast foods that are little more than sugar are healthy or claims that drinking sugary beverages can be "good" for us. On January 9, 2006, *Consumer Reports* reported:

> Recent reports have documented bias in pharmaceutical studies funded by industry. Now, an analysis from Children's Hospital Boston finds a similar phenomenon in scientific articles about nutrition, particularly in studies of beverages.
>
> The analysis—the first systematic one performed on nutrition studies—found that beverage studies funded solely by industry were four to eight times more likely to have conclusions favorable to sponsors' financial interest than were studies with no industry funding.
>
> The findings are published online in the January 9 issue

of the journal *PLoS Medicine*.

David Ludwig, MD, PhD, the study's senior author and director of the Optimal Weight for Life (OWL) program at Children's Hospital Boston, believes that bias in nutrition studies may have far greater effects than bias in pharmaceutical studies [my emphasis]; you can read this study at http://www.consumeraffairs.com/news04/2007/01/food_studies.html.

Free enterprise and capitalism have much to recommend them—scientific and dietary research for clients who expect specific results and are willing to invest money to orchestrate those results is not one of those places.

Another element in the pervasiveness of our unhealthy diet is, literally, propaganda. We're all used to thinking of propaganda as something practiced by Nazis and Communists, but it surrounds us too. Propaganda is little more than the use of covert (and usually deceptive) techniques to sway public opinion or thinking. The key word here is "covert." The propaganda is an idea that is presented in a way that disguises the motive. For instance, claims about the health value of fiber may be broadcast on the evening news. The next day's newspaper might have a story on fiber, and soon stories about the health value of fiber will be appearing all over the internet (usually on blogs sponsored by a laxative maker or another fiber product) as well as other media outlets. What's never revealed to us is that the story probably originated in the public relations department of a pharmaceutical company or industrial food processor which has a lot of worthless industrial waste left over from the manufacturing process that it would rather sell than have to dispose of. If a food manufacturer can sell this worthless and indigestible product at a high price by claiming it has health benefits, why wouldn't he? Well, he might not if he places ethics and decency over profit and career "advancement." However, clearly there are many without the moral "fiber" to do what is right. What gets lost in this process is the consumer, the health of the consumer, and the integrity of the good faith effort to put forward the best and truest information possible.

Nutritionists and physicians are just as susceptible to propaganda, faddism, and orthodoxy as any of us.

As we think about these studies and so-called "healthy food choices" such as fiber, we should also pay attention to human evolution and to the impact that farming and the shift to a grain-based diet has had on the health of human beings. This shift to a grain-based diet has accelerated exponentially in the last 50 years, partly as a result of public policy reinforced by the government and partly because it's much easier to deal with the huge growth in the human population by using grain-based foods as the solution—it's cheap and it helps out the corporate farmers too. We should be asking ourselves questions like these: What did we evolve to eat? What did our ancestors eat? What did our great-grandparents eat? As we ask these questions and search for answers, we should also try to stay as open-minded and objective as possible and not fall into the traps posed by dietary propaganda, food faddism, and dietary correctness.

I want to keep the focus on the importance of looking at the ecology of Inflammatory Bowel Disease, and that means acknowledging the kind of animal humans are as well as our evolutionary history. Evolution usually works with glacial slowness, and as a species we've been around for a long time. To be healthy humans we must eat the diet that we evolved to eat—the diet that is natural to us. The further we travel from the diet of our ancestors—the diet our bodies evolved to consume, process, and derive health from, the more we become susceptible to the constellation of diseases known as "the diseases of civilization." These include such illnesses as diabetes, cancer, Alzheimer's, and heart disease as well as the cluster of auto-immune diseases such as Inflammatory Bowel Disease, Multiple Sclerosis, and Lupus that have seen such dramatic rises in their occurrence during the last forty years. Michael Pollan describes the diet most people in the industrialized world are now eating as "the most radical change to the way humans eat since the discovery of agriculture" (Pollan 10) and goes on to write:

> The plain fact [is] that the chronic diseases that now kill most of us can be traced directly to the industrialization of our food: the rise of highly processed foods and refined grains; the use of chemicals to raise plants and animals in huge monocultures; the superabundance of cheap calories of sugar and fat . . . the narrowing of the biological diversity of the human diet to a tiny handful of staple crops, notably wheat, corn, and soy. These changes have given us the Western diet that we take for granted: lots of processed foods and meat, lots of added fat and sugar, lots of everything (10).

In an almost unbelievable statistic, Pollan notes that only four plants—corn, soy, wheat, and rice—supply two-thirds of the calories Americans consume today. Groves points out that the typical European today gets three quarters of his or her calories from foods that weren't available during the evolution of humans (117).

This fact becomes all the more telling when one considers that Barry Groves points out that 99.99 percent of our genes were in place before the advent of agriculture about 6000 years ago in the Fertile Crescent of the Middle East and that analysis of fossilized human coprolites (excrement) show almost no plant material. Remember that it's only about 6000 years ago that humans began to practice agriculture on a large scale. Yes, strictly-speaking, agriculture dates from about 10,000 years ago, and that's the number usually given in analyses of this topic, but this is when agriculture was first practiced in an isolated and extremely limited and rudimentary way. Most of the evidence from early agricultural sites indicate that the cereal grains being farmed were primarily used as animal feed (we were domesticating animals at the same time) and only began to be used as the basis for a human diet later, after environmental problems made it harder to find sufficient sources of meat and wild plants. It's also good to recognize that agriculture didn't make it to places like northern and western Europe until about

3500 years ago (Ponting 2007). Groves notes that humans have a carnivorous gut, a gut that evolved to digest meat and fat, not plants (196-201). Undigested cereals and grains are the reason so many of us experience bad episodes of gas. These undigested complex carbohydrates are literally fermenting in our guts and giving off gas that we then have to expel. That fermentation is producing and releasing toxins into our bodies, not just making us flatulent.

How did we reach the point where Americans are not only poisoning themselves through what they eat, but where this poisoning is taking place with the encouragement of scientists, corporate "farmers," public policy, and an army of nutritionists. The story is a fascinating cautionary tale which highlights the dangers of both an approach to science, knowledge, and medicine that is fragmented and disjointed, but also of the commercial pressures of science and medicine today. Another issue that rears its ugly head is propaganda and the preponderance of the propaganda technique that the Nazi propagandist, Joseph Goebbels, called the Big Lie.

One of the most important contributors to bad information about diet and nutrition is simply how science and medicine are practiced today. Many different disciplines contribute to our knowledge, but there's no place to tie everything together. Science and medicine are both utterly fragmented today; this fragmentation results in a limited view that makes it almost impossible for most scientists and physicians to practice their disciplines in an integrative way. That's one of the reasons the public is exposed to such a plethora of conflicting information about nutrition. Unfortunately this creates a situation where we learn to distrust our instincts and our ability to filter the conflicting voices and so we turn to the "experts" for our information without realizing that those experts are the ones wearing the blinders that got us into this situation of confusion in the first place.

If a researcher does decide to go against the mainstream, he's probably going to find himself washed ashore and floundering to get back into the professional waters. The way science is practiced today almost demands that one go with the flow if one hopes to be successful. Loren Cordain, a professor at Colorado State University, has pointed out, "There is increasing evidence to indicate that the type of diet recommended in the USDA's food pyramid is discordant with the type of diet humans evolved with over eons of evolutionary experience" (quoted on p. 211 of Groves), but when was the last time you heard a report on information such as this? Researchers such as Loren Cordain and Barry Groves are not concerned specifically with Inflammatory Bowel Disease but with changes in our diet over the last 50 years and the impact these changes, these "modernizations," have had on our health and on the development and proliferation of the diseases of civilization.

Groves argues that the first mistake was made with good intentions but soon got out of hand when about 50 years ago we began to focus on producing and distributing grains and cereals as the primary food for humans as a way of feeding the growing world population. At the same time scientists were hypothesizing a link between cholesterol and heart disease and telling people to avoid saturated animal fats: These two ideas gave us much of the dogma that currently informs the western diet, including the concept that healthy eating means less fat—especially animal fat. The promotion of polyunsaturated vegetable fats as an alternative to animal fats has led to disastrous health consequences. The eating of vegetable oils has turned out to be extremely detrimental to our health (olives are a fruit, not a vegetable) including the atherosclerosis and heart disease they are supposed to prevent. Arthur De Vany notes, "Remember, we consumed no vegetable-based oils at all even as recently as 200 years ago" (44) and reminds us that even olive oil should not be heated too much (beyond 350 degrees) or it will be oxidized and produce free radicals. The result of this move to avoid saturated fats was the replacement of dietary fats with carbohydrates, especially the starches and sugars found in breads, pasta, rice, potatoes, beans, vegetables, and fruit. These carbohydrates became the "preferred" energy sources for our bodies according to nutritionists and many physicians.

Both nutritionists and doctors stressed the point that when thinking about calories, it was important to think only about the quantity of calories a person eats each day and not about the source of those calories. After all, a calorie is a calorie, right—a neutral energy source. Of course, that's a simplification and wrong. Our bodies evolved to eat and take energy from certain kinds of foods, and specifically from eating animals (the whole animal) and animal fats. We have learned, to our dismay, that where the calories come from does matter. It's worth keeping in mind that the incredible rise in obesity, diabetes, and autoimmune diseases taking place today follows this change in our eating habits from carnivores to consumers whose diets are founded on the consumption of lots and lots of carbohydrates and vegetable matter, especially grains and other sources of sugar.

This shifting emphasis in what we should eat was matched by the rapid growth of multi-billion dollar industries to provide low-fat, high-carbohydrate 'healthy' convenience foods to consumers. This was a bonanza for food producers, and the presence of cheap, processed foods has become the foundation of the way most people in industrialized countries now eat.

The shift in our eating habits created another high-growth industry. The multi-billion dollar dieting industry expanded rapidly (and continues to expand) to combat the rising tide of obesity that resulted from the new dogma. This dietary industry does not want you to become slim and stay slim any more than the pharmaceutical industry wants you to get well and stay well. Most "medicines" on the market today create side effects, many of them horrible. One set of symptoms may improve while another is created. It's like privatizing the prison "industry." Any business wants to expand, to grow, to increase its "consumer" base, and to get loyal customers "for life."

Today we have widely-viewed television programs on several continents that involve viewers in the struggles of participants to lose weight under a draconian regime of extreme forced exercise and dieting based around a low-fat diet. The participants are often yelled at while they exercise. The basic philosophy of these shows is one of discovering each participant's *flaw*, the ways in which they are weak and wrong. What's wrong here is the majority of the foods with which we're all surrounded, with which we're constantly tempted. It's not most of America that's "bad." It's the "food products," the mass-produced, chemically altered, additive "enhanced" food stuffs that are wrong—dangerous and wrong. Of course, when one sees these successful dieters a couple of years later, they've usually gained weight because they are still following the dogma that's been pounded into them by nutritionists and the processed food industry. The exceptions are those who have become professional exercisers, personal trainers and the like, who now exercise multiple hours each day to work off all of those carbohydrates they're eating. They may be slim, but surely their bodies are under enormous stress, both from the food they're eating and from the constant, extreme exercise.

This shift in the diet has also been a boon to pharmaceutical products to control cholesterol, appetite, hunger, and blood pressure—all of these consequences of the new dietary regimes that have come to dominate our lives but have little or no good scientific evidence to support them.

The low-fat regimen has become an article of faith. Remember what "dogma" means—strict, unquestioning adherence to unexamined and unproven beliefs. Even though the scientific studies that have been performed to test the efficacy of this diet have not shown it to be effective in reducing cholesterol (a whole different issue), we continue to adhere to it like medieval pilgrims seeking salvation by touching an alleged holy relic.

Michael Pollan states unequivocally:

All of our uncertainties about nutrition should not obscure the plain fact that the chronic diseases that now kill most of us can be traced directly to the industrialization of our food: the rise of highly processed foods and refined grains; the use of chemicals to raise plants and animals in huge monocultures; the superabundance of cheap calories of sugar and fat produced by modern agriculture; and the narrowing of the biological diversity of the human diet to a tiny handful of staple crops, notably wheat, corn, and soy (10).

Both Barry Groves and Michael Pollan explore the role of nutritionists and nutritionism in the rise of the western diet and both argue that the nutritionists are basing their recommendations on bad science (Pollan, 61-80; Groves, 5-6). How can we be expected to eat in a healthy way when we're given "official" advice that is based on bad science and is actually harmful to us—and things are getting worse. Our culture gives us a picture of scientists as ideologically neutral and objective, but of course this isn't true. Scientists are as ideologically impure as any of the rest of us (including me). We see the world through the lenses we have. These lenses are formed through our upbringings in an "information-saturated" media—a media with huge corporate interests. Our lenses are formed during our educations when we're taught the accepted doctrines of the day for doctors, nutritionists, scientists, and other professions, and these lenses are difficult to remove.

Groves points out that today, "Two generations of scientists, nutritionists, dietitians, and doctors [have been] indoctrinated in the 'low-fat' dogma and [the result has been] a consequent decline in the knowledge base" (5). To make things even worse, public health agencies and governments have accepted and supported this faulty approach to eating. Pollan says, "Nutritionism is, in a sense, the official ideology of the Western diet and so cannot be expected to raise radical or searching questions about it" (11). Pollan points out that doing nutrition science is difficult and that the scientific tools available to nutritionists are ill suited to understanding complex systems such as food and diet. Science is, after all, an approach that generally focuses on small-scale things such as molecules that can be analyzed and taken apart. The problem here is the lack of a unifying approach or vision. Another problem Pollan identifies is that "The assumptions of nutritionism—such as the idea that food is not a system but rather the sum of its nutrient parts—pose another set of problems" (61).

This is an issue that goes beyond science. The process of knowing is, by its nature, reductive. We extract things from a world that is truly unknowable in its complexity, and we create a system that attempts to explain that complexity. This is simply the way the mind works and that knowledge progresses—no matter what the discipline. It's as true in the study of literature as it is in science and nutrition. The problem with nutritionism is its lack of integration. Pollan points out that nutritional science typically studies one nutrient at a time, an approach that even some nutritionists acknowledge is flawed. Pollan quotes Marion Nestle, a nutritionist at New York University: "The problem with nutrient-by-nutrient nutrition science is that it takes the nutrient out of the context of the food, the food out of the context of the diet, and the diet out of the context of the lifestyle" (62). But, we don't eat nutrients, we eat food. Food is a system. It contains nutrient calories which developed as a result of the conditions (soil, water, fertilizers, pesticides) under which the food was grown and raised and also includes the additional materials added during further processing (canning, preparation, forming into a cake mix or cracker).

All of this happened in defiance of scientific knowledge. Gary Taubes and Barry Groves both provide devastating critiques of the "science" behind the Western diet and its assumptions.

I think it's fascinating that Inflammatory Bowel Disease and most other auto-immune diseases such as multiple sclerosis and lupus occur at the highest rates among descendants of populations that were among the last to adopt agriculture. Four areas developed agriculture separately and even though there is evidence for the systematic cultivation of grains and other plants as early as 10,000 years ago, agriculture as we know it didn't become part of the human solution to getting enough food until about 6000 years ago in the area known as the Fertile Crescent (Iraq and further south into what is now Israel). It developed in China at about the same time and developed in two different areas of the Americas independently—in Central America and Southern Mexico about 4500 years ago and in the Andes of South America at about the same time. The emphasis in the Middle East was on wheat, in China on rice, in MesoAmerica on corn (maize), and in the Andes on the potato. An agricultural way of life entered southern Europe about 5000 years ago and took longer to become established in northern and western Europe since the climate was wetter and had more rainfall as well as a shorter growing season. Europeans probably settled into an agricultural way of living 2500-3500 years ago. Barry Groves notes, "Diseases of insulin resistance, particularly diabetes, occur with greater frequency in populations that have recently changed dietary habits from hunter-gatherer to western cereal grain-based regimes" (215).

We have allowed ourselves to become subjects in what is essentially an exercise in the evolutionary principle of adaptation and how effectively a species can adapt to a huge and rapid change in its environment—its ecology. We're experimenting with how a species adapts to a rapidly changing diet, and the enormous increases in the diseases of civilization powerfully show us that we're having a lot of trouble adapting. I don't know about you, but I'm not willing to be the subject in an experiment like this.

Our species evolved over millennia and agriculture is, in evolutionary terms, not only a radically new diet, but a radically different diet that our bodies have not had much time to adapt to. We are designed to eat like hunters and gatherers, and that doesn't mean hunting and gathering the corn puffs and snack foods in the grocery store.

Chapter 7
Carrageenan: A Major Villain

I'm convinced that carrageenan was created by the evolutionary equivalent of the devil, and that it entered the human food supply with the aid of his demon Beelzebub. Unfortunately, this destructive additive has become ubiquitous in the food chain—especially in processed foods. If you make only one change in your diet, it should be to do everything in your power to avoid this "natural" food additive.

Here's a fun fact: carrageenan is used in the laboratory to induce ulcerative colitis and inflammatory bowel disease in rats. That pretty much sums it up, but a detailed exploration of this additive from hell might help understand it a bit more.

Carrageenan is extracted from red seaweed and is found in a wide variety of processed foods. It's easy to find on labels, so if you see this item as an ingredient, avoid the product. That's right—put it back on the shelf. Carrageenan is also widely used in restaurants, however, and there it can be more difficult to avoid. A number of different kinds of carrageenan are used in food processing. For instance, one type (Kappa-carrageenan) is used widely in breading and batters because it helps things gel. Another kind of carrageenan (Lambda carrageenan) doesn't have gelling properties, but is used to bind the products in sweet doughs together since it helps these doughs retain moisture and improves the texture of the product. A third type (Iota carrageenan) is used with fruit. To sum up, carrageenan is used to thicken things (buttermilk, soups, pudding, maple syrup, ice cream), to help liquids stay mixed together without separating (half and half, salad dressing,) to "improve" a food's texture (making it thicker or chewier—breads, pastries, puddings), and to stabilize foods (to help sugar, sorbet, or ice cream from developing crystals).

You'll find this everywhere: whipping cream, half and half, ice cream sorbet, yogurt, sour cream, bread, doughnuts, cookies, cakes, pies, milkshakes, sweetened condensed milk, sauces, gravies, beer, patés, processed meats, toothpaste, candy, soy milk, baby formula, and diet soda. This list doesn't even begin to address the variety of commercial uses for carrageenan. It's even found in "personal lubricants" and shampoos.

You'll also find it promoted in "natural foods" as a vegetarian or vegan alternative to gelatin and in "low-fat" products to make the food creamier once the fats have been removed. Carrageenan has been used as an additive for hundreds (perhaps thousands) of years. In fact, some of the Irish who immigrated to the United States in the 19th century made their living by collecting seaweed off the coast of New England and selling that seaweed for processing into carrageenan. Often carrageenan is promoted as a "natural" product, but keep in mind that the solvents used to extract carrageenan are so potent that they would remove the skin from your hands. I suppose one could call this "natural," but only if you're also willing to extend that label to MSG (extracted from rice) or Aspartame (extracted from petroleum). That still doesn't mean it's good for us. In the past one of the uses of carrageenan was topically, as an ointment, to treat venereal disease. Yum, yum.

Remember that humans only widely adopted agriculture six to eight thousand years ago, or, in some cultures, in the last 100-200 years, and that our bodies are still trying to deal with the shock of our shift from a diet based on meat, fresh "vegetables," and fruit (what we could hunt and gather) to a diet based on cereal grains, potatoes, and other complex carbohydrates. I don't know about you, but I'm not willing to sacrifice my health in order to participate in a government-sponsored, corporate-controlled evolutionary experiment.

Dr. Andrew Weil points out that the results of a study published in October 2001 suggest that carrageenan causes both ulcerations and cancers of the gastrointestinal tract (http://www.drweil.com/drw/u/id/QAA44833). The researcher who made the connection between carrageen and cancer is Joanne Tobacman, an assistant professor of clinical internal medicine at the University of Iowa College of Medicine. Dr. Tobacman published her findings in the article, "Review of Harmful Gastrointestinal Effects of Carrageenan in Animal Experiments," in the October 2001 issue of *Environmental Health Perspective*. The food industry went into a major public relations spin mode after this publication, and if you do a search for carrageenan on the internet, you will find a plethora of articles reassuring you that this additive is harmless and that research has disproven Dr. Tobacman's research. Please don't let yourself be conned. Remember that the processed food industry is focused on profits and not on your health.

Ray Peat (http://raypeat.com/articles/nutrition/carrageenan.shtml) points out that carrageenan has been recognized as a dangerous allergen since the 1940s, and is used "to produce inflammatory tumors (granulomas), immunodeficiency, arthritis, other inflammations." Peat also notes that diseases such as Crohn's have been increasing over the last fifty years as carrageenan has become a more common food additive in industrialized countries.

If you're doubting me, just read the introduction to a 2008 study by Sumit Bhattacharyya, Alip Borthakur, Pradeep K. Dudeja, and Joanne K. Tobacman from the Department of Medicine at the University of Illinois at Chicago:

> The common food additive carrageenan (CGN) has been widely used for decades in models of intestinal inflammation

to test the effects of pharmacological interventions for treatment of inflammatory bowel disease and to study the inflammatory response. Dozens of studies in animals have demonstrated profound effects of CGN on the intestinal mucosa, producing ulcerations and neoplasms (*The Journal of Nutrition*, 2008, p. 469).

The food industry and carrageenan producers have mounted a public relations campaign, and websites often defend carrageenan as healthy. The webstite carrageenan.info states, that the JECFA (Joint FAO/WHO Expert Committee on Food Additives) found carrageenan safe for human consumption since the levels of carrageenan used to induce gastrointestinal problems in rats was higher than humans consume and concludes that carrageenan does not pose a threat to human health. Other websites produce different rationales for carrageenan as acceptable—for example, because it's "natural." This is a word to be cautious about. Lots of food producers include the word "natural" in their advertising because it's a positive word for most people and shorts circuits our critical thinking about whether or not something is actually good for us. It's natural—it must be good, right? I try to remember one of the things the late comic George Carlin said: Dogshit's natural, but it's just not real good food. The main thing to remember is that the websites promoting carrageenan as neutral or even positive are almost always linked to carrageenan producers or to the processed food industry.

More and more people are realizing the dangers of carrageenan. This was posted on healthnowmedical.com/blog/2011/05/16/is-carrageenan-a-safe-food-additive/ on May 16, 2011 by Dr. Vikkii Petersen:

> Carrageenan is a newer additive, relatively speaking. It is made from seaweed, and for that reason I always considered it to be rather innocent—I was mistaken. Apparently, experimentally, it's used as an agent to induce intense inflammation in experimental animals. A study done several years ago found that when carrageenan is injected into

animals along with a cancer-causing chemical, tumors appeared more rapidly and in higher numbers than in animals injected with the carcinogen alone (2011).

I know that carrageenan has strongly negative effects on me, and I avoid it completely. I will see symptoms within 24 hours if I accidentally consume this additive although they usually disappear quickly after accidental consumption. However, before I started smoking to control ulcerative colitis, I would bleed **the next day** after eating carrageenan. Often that bleeding rapidly turned into a full-blown flare. Carrageenan has almost killed me—repeatedly. It's almost impossible to avoid this additive completely if you eat out since it's a component of so many processed foods. Do everything you can to keep consumption of this carrageenan at the lowest possible level—ideally at a level of no consumption. I rarely eat out anymore because at home I have complete say over what goes on my plate, but when traveling eating out is often obligatory. My solution is to avoid anything "creamy"—sauces, gravies, and soups. I squint at the labels on the tiny containers of cream or half and half to see if carrageenan is listed as an ingredient, and if it is, I drink my tea or coffee without cream. I skip dessert.

Perhaps one day the agricultural and food processing industries will be held accountable for their crimes against humanity, their endangerment of the public, and the serious disease and even death which they contribute to and at times cause. Meanwhile, we need to be well-informed, vigilant, and prudent consumers. As much as possible, we should try to ensure that our diet consists of high-quality products—preferably, fresh, organic, and local foods.

Chapter 8
The Fiber Problem

Dietary fiber is another of the great cons of the processed food industry. Today fiber is presented as not only something to be used as a supplemental part of the diet but as a necessary and beneficial part of everyone's diet. As Konstantin Monastyrsky points out in *Fiber Menace: The Truth about Fiber's Role in Diet Failure, Constipation, Hemorrhoids, Irritable Bowel Syndrome, Ulcerative Colitis, Crohn's Disease, and Colon Cancer* (2008):

> Fiber is a relatively new phenomenon in human nutrition. As little as a few hundred years ago—an eye blink on the evolutionary timeline—people couldn't consume fiber because there were no industrial mills, no stainless steel grinders, and no high-temperature ovens to convert (process) what is really livestock feed into foodstuff fit for human consumption (9).

What we think of as dietary fiber comes in two forms: soluble and insoluble. Soluble fiber absorbs water and becomes a gel-like substance in the intestinal tract where it is fermented (producing gas) by bacteria. Insoluble fiber is simply an indigestible product that creates bulk in the intestines and is not fermented. Soluble fiber is found in all plant foods, but is especially high in beans and peas, vegetables such as broccoli and carrots, fruits and berries, and cereals like oats and rye. Psyllium husks (often found in products designed to fight constipation) are also a source of soluble fiber. Insoluble fiber is found in whole grain foods, nuts, seeds, some vegetables such as cauliflower and zucchini, and in cereal brans. Fiber is really nothing more than the parts of plants that resist human digestive enzymes. Remember that soluble fiber is "digested" by a process of fermentation—this is where flatulence or gas comes from. If you aren't fermenting foods in your intestines, you won't be passing gas. We're all going to get some fiber in our diets from the plant foods we eat, and eating fiber in amounts that are suited to our evolutionary history is useful since small amounts of soluble fiber slow the digestive process and allow our intestines to absorb nutrients, vitamins, and minerals. We can get all of the fiber we need through eating some vegetables or a little fruit or a handful of nuts. This can also be useful in regulating blood sugar. The problems with fiber arise when we eat too much of it—especially in the insoluble form.

Dietary fiber didn't really become part of the "nutrition" landscape until the 1970s. We might understand the marketing and media push of fiber consumption more clearly if we remembered that "dietary fiber" is little more than a way for agribusiness to profit from a substance that has traditionally been disposed of as a waste product of agricultural processes. Corporate agribusiness is brilliant at finding ways to market useless, even harmful, products and byproducts and profiting from the results. This is often based on propaganda the industrial food manufacturers produce and, indeed, the techniques of these food manufacturers is an example of propaganda at its finest. What's inexcusable, however, is that the nutritional experts of our culture have bought into this propaganda. Goebbels, Hitler's Minister of Propaganda might have admired the marketing of chaff, or fiber, as an example of his most beloved propaganda technique—the "big lie"—but I doubt that even Goebbels could have foreseen a situation such as the nutritional one currently existing in industrialized countries. Adolf Hitler actually coined the expression, "the big lie," in his 1925 book, *Mein Kampf* as a definition for a lie so huge that no one would believe that someone "could have the impudence to distort the truth so infamously."

A number of researchers have pointed out the uselessness—the destructiveness—of dietary fiber for humans. Barry Groves uses the image of fiber as similar to putting sandpaper in our intestines. Of course, this irritant causes our bowels to move. Too much fiber can cause a number of miserable side effects such as, ironically, increased constipation and increased flatulence.

For those suffering from Inflammatory Bowel Disease fiber can be a disaster. If you've bought into the fiber propaganda produced by the media and the food industry, two writers who provide succinct and clear histories of the introduction of fiber into the western diet are Gary Taubes in *Good Calories, Bad Calories* (2007, pp. 122-135) and Barry Groves in *Trick and Treat* (2008, pp. 118-128). Both of these writers also provide an extensive list of sources on how the "fiber hypothesis" developed and was propagated in western culture as well as a number of sources (including large studies by leading medical schools) that have **disproved** the idea that fiber has health benefits. This is the part of the fiber story that has NOT been presented to us.

In his book Taubes discusses fiber in the context of the early 70s and the concern over heart disease and points out, "The fiber hypothesis captured the public's nutritional consciousness by virtue of the messianic efforts of a single investigator, a former missionary surgeon named Denis Burkitt, who proposed that this indigestible roughage was a requisite component of a healthy diet" (124). Burkitt and a colleague, Alec Walker, published an article in *The Lancet*, which started the process of introducing fiber into the public consciousness and to the place it holds as unquestioned "law" in the mainstream dietary guidelines and advice dispensed today. Burkitt originally associated lack of fiber with appendicitis, diverticulitis, and colon cancer, but quickly extended his hypothesis about the necessity of fiber in diet to a number of other diseases and chronic conditions.

The media quickly picked up this story about fiber and its alleged benefits for heart disease. Taubes points to 1972 articles in *The Washington Post* (which called fiber 'the tonic for our time') and *Reader's Digest* that helped shift public thinking about fiber and notes that within a year such giants of the breakfast food industry as General Mills and Kellogg immediately began pushing bran and fiber as heart-healthy foods. This push continues today.

Taubes goes on to note that over the last twenty-five years, there has been no evidence to support the fiber hypothesis while

> there has been a steady accumulation of evidence refuting the notion that a fiber-deficient diet causes colon cancer, polyps, or diverticulitis, let alone any other disease of civilization. The pattern is precisely what would be expected of a hypothesis that simply isn't true: the larger and more rigorous the trials set up to test it, the more consistently negative the evidence (132).

Taubes points to the Nurses Health Study (1994) conducted by the Harvard School of Public Health which concluded that the consumption of fiber, fruits, and vegetables is unrelated to the risk of colon cancer. Taubes also cites the Dietary Modification Trial of the Women's Health Initiative (2006, studied 49,000 women) as confirming that eating more fiber (whole grains, vegetables, fruits) "had no beneficial effect on colon cancer, nor did it prevent heart disease or breast cancer or induce weight loss" (132-33). In spite of this, the media continues to push the fiber hypothesis (Taubes cites a number of examples, 134-5).

The British researcher Barry Groves devastates the fiber hypothesis in his book *Trick and Treat*. Groves emphasizes how quickly the commercial food industry took up the fiber hypothesis as well as the reasons they were so quick to begin pushing fiber:

> bran has a far higher fibre content than vegetables and bran was a practically worthless by-product of the milling process

which, until then, had been thrown away. Bran is quite inedible—there is no known enzyme in the human body that can digest it; nevertheless, backed by Burkitt's fibre hypothesis, commercial interests could now promote it as a valuable food. Virtually overnight, it became a highly priced profit maker (119).

Groves further points out that bran is nothing more than the outer covering of grains and every civilization in history has developed methods of separating the wheat from the chaff so that they wouldn't have to eat it—that's what bran is—the chaff—an agricultural waste product.

Far from being healthy, fiber can actually be extremely destructive to health. Groves points to studies in the mid 1980s which found dietary fiber to **increase** the risk of colon cancer (119), as well as a British study in 1990 which found arguments that fiber could help irritable bowel syndrome or diverticulosis and colon cancer to be unfounded (120). Other studies reached similar conclusions in 1995 and 1996. These are in addition to the studies that Taubes mentions.

Groves also points out that since fiber speeds the movement of food through the digestive system, fiber can inhibit the absorption of "such nutrients as zinc, iron, calcium, phosphorus, magnesium, energy, proteins, fats, and vitamins, A, D, E, and K" (124). As a result this can contribute to deficiency diseases and poor nutrition. Insoluble fiber such as oat bran "can cause numerous problems with digestion and assimilation, leading to mineral deficiencies, irritable bowel syndrome, and auto-immune conditions such as Crohn's Disease" (126).

Groves reports on how fiber works to move things through the gut. Interestingly, this process wasn't made clear until 2006 after scientists at the Medical College of Georgia studied it. Fiber works because the rough, bulky bran scratches and tears cells in the gut wall. Cell biologist, Dr. Paul L. McNeill describes it this way: "this banging and tearing increases the level of lubricating mucus. It's a good thing" (127). Can it really be a good thing to apply the equivalent of sandpaper to the delicate lining of the intestines? Clearly, no.

Groves reminds us that before the mid-20th century, dietary fiber was regarded as harmful. For people who had gut disorders the recommendation was to avoid bran and adopt a low fiber diet. After Burkitt published his article, many physicians began to put both Irritable Bowel Syndrome and Inflammatory Bowel Disease under the same umbrella as colon cancer (with no real evidence to support the recommendation) and to endorse Burkitt's recommendations of high fiber to avoid colon cancer. A number of studies have shown no convincing effect of any benefit at all of bran on symptoms of IBS. In 1987 a study was done to test fiber's efficacy with IBS. The results were that people who consumed bran were worse off than people who didn't. "The weight of all the evidence suggests that bran, wholemeal bread and wholemeal cereals are more likely to cause IBS than they are to cure it. Also, because it is indigestible, bran ferments in the gut and can induce or exacerbate flatulence, distension and abdominal pain. And it is the same story with diverticular disease" (355). If you're passing gas frequently and if that gas is offensive, there's something wrong with your digestive processes. One of the best things you can do to eliminate the symptoms of Inflammatory Bowel Disease and Irritable Bowel Syndrome is to detox your gut and minimize the process of carbohydrate fermentation that's producing that gas.

Of course there is a great deal of information that supports the use of fiber, but try to approach this information with a degree of skepticism. Be especially wary of the advice on fiber that comes from websites: Here's an example from http://www.healthcastle.com/ibd-diet.shtml

> Inflammatory Bowel Disease, IBD, including Crohn's Disease and ulcerative colitis, is an inflammation of the intestines. These diseases cause the intestines to form ulcers and become inflamed, scarred, and easy to bleed. . . . Diet

and nutrition is very important in IBD management to prevent malnutrition and extreme weight loss.

This website then provides the following diet advice: "Eat a high fiber diet when IBD is under control. Click here for a list of high fiber foods. Some patients find cooking and steaming the vegetables more tolerable than eating them raw." Please remember that dietary fiber provides absolutely NO nutritional value to anyone who eats it—there's an immediate contradiction here, and the danger of actually exacerbating the existing condition through attempts to help it. Remember Barry Groves' image of fiber functioning like sandpaper on the lining of the colon? The website does have the decency to say: "During a flare up, however, limit high fiber foods and follow a low fiber diet or even a low residue diet to give the bowel a rest and minimize symptoms." Most of the websites that explore fiber need to be approached cautiously. Some seem to be produced by propagandists for the industrial food processors while others propagandize for the benefits of vegetarianism or veganism. All of them have bought into the dietary orthodoxy and unexamined assumptions that dominate today's nutritional landscapes.

Why would anyone suffering from IBD take the chance on dietary fiber whether she is in the middle of a flare or not? One might as well scoop up spoonfuls of carrageenan when symptom free. Anyone who has endured a flare up of this disease will do anything possible to avoid a flare and avoiding a high fiber diet should be at the top of the list.

Be skeptical of anyone selling supplements or promoting a product that will heal your IBD while putting money in their pockets by selling their own products and dietary supplements. Natural medicines and herbal remedies are not regulated by the government, and far too many of these are little more than vicious schemes that prey on an individual's desperate desire for healing.

When thinking about fiber, remember that it costs practically nothing, and the chances are that it would just be thrown away as a waste product if it weren't being used to bulk up foods and profits. It seems so profoundly and fundamentally unethical to profit from the endangerment of the public health, but as we all know, it's common for health to take a backseat to profits. There really are no positive benefits to be had from adding any fiber to the diet beyond that in the fruits and vegetables we normally eat.

One source of fiber to be extremely careful about is brown rice. Brown rice is nothing more than rice that hasn't had the outer covering (the chaff) removed. Brown rice is often promoted as a healthy, fiber-rich, "natural" food, and I have found sites devoted to inflammatory bowel disease that recommend eating brown rice. After carrageenan, brown rice has been the worst producer of flares for me. Eating brown rice has led to a number of significant flares, which would often start the very day after consuming brown rice.

I've been in complete remission for over five years as a result of diet and the use of nicotine. However, if I unwittingly eat a product that contains brown rice or high amounts of fiber, I experience diarrhea (although no longer bloody and not mucus-filled), gas, and other symptoms of intestinal distress. I'm sure that if I consumed these products on a regular basis, I would rapidly begin to experience the traditional symptoms of Inflammatory Bowel Disease again. Fiber is not something we evolved to eat. We don't have the same kind of teeth or digestive tract that herbivores such as cows have, and we shouldn't be eating the same kinds of foods that they eat. Avoiding excess fiber is one of the best things you can to do heal and to improve your general health.

Chapter 9
Sugar and Sweeteners

Talk about a rat's nest. Sugar has become more and more central to the Western diet. Werner L. Knoepp notes that in the year 1700 the average sugar consumption of an American was four pounds a year. This figure had increased to eighteen pounds a year by 1800. Today, the average American consumes 180 pounds of sugar each year (2011). Think about this for a minute—that's half a pound of sugar a day, or the equivalent of almost a five pound bag of sugar each week. Knoepp notes that most infant formulas have as much sugar as a full can of soda. Sugar is added to practically all fruit juices and also to processed foods such as peanut butter and ketchup as well as to such products as yogurt, crackers, and bread. Even "low fat" foods designed to help people lose weight are packed with sugar. In fact, usually the low fat version of a food is far less healthy and should be avoided because of increased sugar content and other additives in these foods. Excess sugar consumption has been linked not only to obesity but to diabetes, heart disease, increased cholesterol levels, and metabolic syndrome.

Michael Pollan notes that

One of the most momentous changes in the American diet since 1909 (when the USDA first began keeping track) has been the increase in the percentage of calories coming from sugar, from 13 percent to 20 percent. Add to that the percentage of calories coming from carbohydrates (roughly 40 percent, or ten servings, nine of which are refined) and Americans are consuming a diet that is at least half sugars in one form or another (112).

Today, sugar is found in all sorts of places it shouldn't be. I was stunned to see dextrose added to hamburger meat being sold in grocery stores. Most people eating the Western diet are in a more or less constant state of insulin overload. Sugar is problematic whether one is talking about sucrose, fructose, corn syrup, high fructose corn syrup, or honey. The Specific Carbohydrate diet, for instance, forbids all sugars except honey since honey is a monosaccharide carbohydrate and so easier to digest. Other dietary approaches say to avoid honey as well.

Unfortunately, much misinformation about sugar is floating through our information landscape (most of it funded by the sugar industry). As I mentioned earlier, in my research I even found one book that recommended that people suffering from Inflammatory Bowel Disease should eat sugar. De Lamar Gibbons' book, *The Self-Help Way to Treat Colitis and Other IBS Conditions*, is based around avoiding fructose, the sugar found in fruit. He identifies this particular sugar as the primary culprit in the disease. He then goes on to say that he sees no problems with sucrose—common, refined table sugar (86) and actually lists sugar (as well as white bread) as the first of his "friendly foods" for those with inflammatory bowel disease. He does suggest staying away from corn sweeteners since these have some fructose. It's worth noting that high fructose corn syrup has become the most common sugar added to processed foods and sodas today. In contradiction to books that take a critical look at the Western diet from an evolutionary perspective, Gibbons writes, "The human body was designed to use starch as its principal fuel source. Starch is concentrated glucose" (88), and Gibbons goes on to make such statements as "...one may drink diet soda pop all day with no untoward effects to the bowel" (90). Not only is this statement untrue, it's dangerous.

The Specific Carbohydrate Diet, an otherwise helpful and thoughtful approach to diet, suggests that it's fine to use saccharin as a sugar substitute. Saccharin is never "fine."

This kind of information is dangerous. A number of writers have linked sugar consumption to the carbohydrate hypothesis, which postulates that a diet high in sugar and carbohydrates leads to the so-called diseases of civilization which include diabetes, chronic heart disease, and autoimmune diseases. All of these illnesses have increased dramatically since western culture has shifted to a carbohydrate-rich, refined-grain diet. Artificial sweeteners include acesulfame-k, sorbitol, aspartame, neotame, and saccharine. These "sweeteners" are among the **worst things** anyone can eat. Some of the potential problems that have been identified with these artificial sweeteners include cancer, headaches, panic attacks, mood changes, visual hallucinations, manic episodes, dizziness, temper outbursts, seizure, nervousness, insomnia, shrunken thymus glands, enlarged liver, enlarged kidneys, and depression. Some of these sweeteners are fat insoluble and so can collect in the fat cells of the body until they become toxic. Along with sugar, artificial sweeteners may play a role in Metabolic Syndrome. Unfortunately these artificial sweeteners show up in many places where one wouldn't expect them such as in vitamin and herb supplements, breath mints, yogurt, cocoa mixes, and even in toothpaste and mouthwashes. This is another time when it pays to read labels. Like carrageenan, artificial sweeteners have insidiously made their way into many products, and anyone suffering from inflammatory bowel disease should do everything possible to avoid them. Ideally, no one would ever consume another drop of artificial sweetener—ever. They're that harmful.

Humans seem to have a "sweet tooth" built into our system, but this comes from an evolutionary history during which honey was the only "sweet" available to us, and honey was seasonal, rare, and difficult to obtain for almost all of our history. Our bodies really aren't designed to use sugar except on rare occasions and in small amounts. We've had much less time to adapt evolutionarily to sugar than to grains—only a few hundred years. Some research has found that sugar is addictive in the same way that an opiate or nicotine is addictive. It's possible to break the sugar addiction, and you will feel much better and take a huge step toward healing inflammatory bowel disease if you can break this addiction.

The best alternative to sugar is stevia, a plant with a sweet taste. It's an herb like basil or parsley, and has virtually no calories or carbohydrates. Honey, if used in moderation, is another way to satisfy one's sweet tooth. Maple syrup, coconut sugar, and agave sugar have also become increasingly popular as sweeteners—especially in products marketed toward those who want to eat "natural" foods. It might be worth exploring these, but agave sugar is a much more concentrated way of delivering sweetness than even common refined table sugar.

I avoid sugar as much as possible. I always read labels carefully. If I have any indication that things aren't right in my bowels, I make sure that I cut out all possible sources of sugar immediately. It was during the time that I followed the Specific Carbohydrate Diet for about two years that I developed a cautious approach to sugars. After my pancreas shut down and I had to use insulin for a while, I became even more careful with sugar. I was lucky to discover *Dr. Bernstein's Diabetes Solution* early in my dealings with diabetes, and like many of the other writers who have been willing to look at things for themselves and not through the lens of current nutritional dogma, he advocates a very low carbohydrate diet. Again, his book is the single best one I found for diabetes and is also excellent for a general approach to low-carbohydrate eating.

Chapter 10
Soy

It's hard to decide which is the greatest nutritional hoax perpetrated on people trying to stay healthy and alive on the standard western diet: fiber or soy. Both soy and fiber have had disastrous consequences on our health, yet we're encouraged to make them a larger and larger part of our diet since they're supposed to be healthy for us. They have certainly been healthy for the profits of the processed food industry even though soy used to be listed in the United States Department of Agriculture Handbook (in 1913) as an industrial product rather than as a food!

Among the claims for soy that currently spread through the mass media and the WorldWideWeb are that it is a "near perfect food," that it "can provide an ideal source of protein, lower cholesterol, protect against cancer and heart disease, reduce menopausal symptoms, and prevent osteoporosis" (www.naturalness.com retrieved May 28, 2011). So many fallacies surround soy that it's hard to know where to begin. These fallacies include the idea that soy has long been a major part of the Asian diet. It hasn't been—even today it contributes a very small amount of the diet in Asia and what it does contribute is almost exclusively in a fermented form (unlike the non-fermented form that it usually takes in the industrial diet). The only way soy should ever be consumed is after it has been fermented in such fermented soy products as natto, tempeh, miso, soy sauce, or tamari. Prior to fermentation, soy is toxic.

Barry Groves focuses on the negative effects of soy on the thyroid and its function but notes that there is a major debate about whether or not soy is healthy for humans (156). At first glance soy seems like a beneficial food and one that could easily serve as a meat substitute. Soy is low in carbohydrates and high in protein and as a result is used in a wider and wider range of foods from breakfast cereals to salad dressing. I've even found soy lecithin (a waste product that results from the processing of soy) in Celestial Seasonings Teas, specifically the Honey-Vanilla Chamomile. Soy lecithin, like carrageenan, works as an emulsifier to hold things like candy bars and bread together. Soy is also increasingly promoted for those who want to eat a healthy, organic diet, for vegetarians and vegans, and for those who are trying to lose weight.

Some of the problems Groves identifies with soy include the toxins associated with it such as protease inhibitors which block some of the enzymes needed for protein digestion and as a result create gastric problems; the poor digestion of protein; the inhibited absorption of important minerals in the gut, and inhibited thyroid activity. Soy also contains phytoestrogens and isoflavones, which imitate the action of estrogen—the female sex hormone—just what every man wants to be putting into his body. While it is obvious that men do not need a bunch of "estrogen" in their bodies, a moment's reflection might make it clear that most women probably don't need a lot of extra female hormones either, particularly if they are pregnant or breast-feeding and will therefore pass those hormones on to their infants. A variety of studies have linked soy consumption to fertility disorders and infertility as well as to increased cancer and leukemia in children (Groves, 160).

Soy has long been a part of Asian diets, but the soy that people traditionally eat is fermented in a process that destroys most of the toxins associated with this legume. Non-fermented soy products (and this includes tofu) still contain these toxins. In addition to tofu and bean curd, products such as infant formula, soy milk, protein powders, meat substitutes, and garden burgers also contain unfermented soy. Almost all of the ways soy is used in modern industrial food production involve its unfermented varieties, and it's becoming harder and harder to find food products that don't have soy in them.

Groves points out that soy milk was originally a waste product of tofu production. Isn't it fascinating how these waste products such as soy milk and bran are now promoted by the food industry as healthy foods? They're even expensive. I'm sure these guys could find a way to turn lint and earwax into "healthy" additions to our diets if there were profit to be made. Soy milk has become an important part of the diets of many people who are lactose intolerant as well as of many people who truly want to live in an ethically responsible way and leave the smallest footprint possible on the earth. Don't be taken in by the propaganda of either the processed food industry or the natural foods industry. They do not have your best interests at heart.

Soy also inhibits the absorption of zinc—a mineral that is crucial for the development of the brain and nervous system. A number of parents have reported infants developing ulcerative colitis and intestinal bleeding after they were fed soy-based formula. An infant who consumes only soy-based formula receives the equivalent (in phytoestrogens) of five birth control pills each day (www.naturalness.com retrieved May 28, 2011). Groves cites a 25-year study of individuals who consumed a diet high in tofu in middle-age then having brain damage in later life (Groves, note 12, p 159). This deterioration included brain atrophy and cognitive impairment no matter how small the level of tofu consumption.

Soy is especially problematic for men and children. Practically all mass-produced breads today include soy flour or soy lecithin. One clear place where this may be observed is in the lowered age of puberty for girls—now at an average of 10 years old.

Phytoestrogen, which occurs in high levels in soy, reduces testosterone in men. This can reduce a man's sex drive and may be associated with breast cancer in men. The Global Healing Center found that the isoflavones in soy milk can decrease the amount of sperm produced by men by as much as forty percent.

A number of sources are available that explore the "dark side" of soy—the side that is rarely presented to the public. One good source from the web is www.westonaprice.org; probably the best book exploring the larger dietary and health issues associated with soy is *The Whole Soy Story: The Dark Side of America's Favorite Health Food* (2005) by Kaayla T. Daniel. Daniel provides a history of soy in both Asia and the West, looks at how soy is used, and explores the many dangers that soy poses to health. She also has a great chapter on how soy has been spun as a health food. Most of her book is devoted to the negative health impacts of soy. One excellent chapter contains a description of the waste product soy lecithin ("industrial sludge," in her words) and the omnipresence of this industrial waste in our food as an emulsifier.

What about soy's relationship to IBD? It's definitely something to think about, although it's hard to find information on soy and inflammatory bowel disease that isn't straight from the soy industry or the so-called "natural foods" industry. One woman who posted on www.revolution health.com/forums/digestive/ulcerative-colitis/81550 (retrieved May 28, 2011) said that two of her three young daughters developed colitis that was completely caused by soy. This poster's youngest daughter had blood in her diaper the day after she was given soy-based formula. They immediately took the soy out of her diet and no blood has appeared since. Her older daughter was on soy formula for eight months before blood appeared. This daughter had a colonoscopy which confirmed ulcerative colitis. The colitis improved slowly after soy was removed from her diet, but according to the mother's reports the blood did not disappear until she went off sulfasalazine. The child's doctors insisted that soy had nothing to do with the colitis and recommended she go back on soy a year later. Two days later blood had reappeared even though she had been in remission for a year and was still taking sulfasalazine. This is hardly a scientific sample, but one of the things I've learned in dealing with inflammatory bowel disease is to trust my experience and the experience and observations of others. It's hard to imagine a scientist or physician who would pay as close attention to their subjects as a mother would. This mother's experience was not an isolated one. Many parents report their children having negative symptoms after beginning soy-based formula. The evidence is so damning that soy-based infant formula should be avoided. Goat's milk is incredibly healthy and might be an excellent choice for children or others who have trouble with cow's milk.

Scientific research supports not using soy-based infant formula. *The Journal of Pediatrics* published an article in September 1977 (Volume 91, issue 3, pp 404-407) by the physicians Thomas C. Halpin, William J. Byrne, and Marvin Ament titled "Colitis, persistent diarrhea, and soy protein intolerance" which found a link between colitis and soy protein based formula. Biopsies in this study found acute ulcerative colitis, and the article recommended that if a baby had persistent and bloody diarrhea and was drinking soy formula, the formula should be removed from the diet. Of course this was in 1977—before we had all been propagandized that this health food was good for us.

A study at the University of Arkansas Medical School conducted in 1994 by A. W. Burks, H. B. Casteel and others found that thirty-three percent of infants given powdered soy formula experienced proctitis or colitis and that thirty percent of infants given liquid soy formula experienced proctitis or colitis.

Unfortunately, many sources on the web and in print continue to recommend soy. For example on the website "Wellness Self-Care & Relationship Resources Colitis/Crohn's (www.carolynchambersclark.com/id39.html) you will find advice that follows most of the "natural" approaches to "health" including:

"Focus your food around soy (soy milk, soy burgers, tofu, tempeh, soy cheese, soy meats), some fresh fruit and loads of green leafy vegetables."

Use your common sense and learn from the experience of others and not the propaganda of industrial food processors and those who are convinced that because it's a vegetable protein soy will be the salvation of the world. I'm an environmentalist and regularly wear Birkenstocks and Earth shoes, but I also want to think for myself, and I don't want 20 to 30 bloody stools a day because I can't give up the brainwashed belief that eating soy is "good" for me and for the planet.

Chapter 11
Cereal Grains, Gluten, and the Specific Carbohydrate Diet

One of the themes that has run throughout this book has been the issue of diet. Frequently, physicians and those who work with inflammatory bowel disease tell us that diet is not related to developing inflammatory bowel disease although they will often acknowledge that specific foods might exacerbate a flare. Another theme that I've developed throughout this book is the idea of illness, diet, treatment, and information as ecologies or systems that interlock and create the world in which we find ourselves. This is a world that we need to learn to reinhabit.

Cereal grains and the gluten that accompanies most of them are, along with soy and sugar, the linchpins of the food ecology we currently inhabit—these foods provide the cornerstone of the Standard American diet today. We are propagandized to accept that it is a healthy diet, propagandized by our governments and public policy as well as by the nutritionism establishment, the medical establishment, and the pharmaceutical industrial food complex. We are also made to feel immoral and irresponsible if our food choices aren't built on these foods. Too often today people view food choices and other personal choices such as the decision to smoke or not to smoke through a prism of morality. Of course, one could argue that there is an ethical dimension to eating. Factory farming of animals is cruel and little more than a form of torture for the animals who endure it. However, the monocultural approach to growing plants is also horribly destructive to the environment and environmental systems. We live in a world where humanity has essentially adopted a totalitarian attitude toward everything that isn't human (and sometimes even toward other humans). Factory farming of animals and monocultural exploitation of miles and miles of land are simply the most brutal examples of this totalitarian approach to the world. Totalitarianism infects the ecologies of food, medicine, nutritionism, pharmaceuticals, and information. This is wrong. Eating is not a matter of morality. Eating is something we all do and something that too many of us have little control over—especially if we live in an urban area and shop in a traditional grocery store. We do not become virtuous people or moral people or immoral people as a result of the foods we eat or the treatments we use to control a disease. Most of us have little choice about this.

One of the things that is missing from the current discussion of health and eating is a recognition of the evolutionary history of humanity. Our ancestors were not vegans or even vegetarians. Humans evolved as omnivores, but our digestive system is not designed to handle cereals or many of the other things we routinely put into them today. It's essential that we move away from a false notion of what our ancestors were like. They ate meat and fats, lots of fat—as often as they could and as much as they could; they ate fruit when it was in season. They ate lots of leaves and berries and probably some roots and mushrooms—they may even have chased other animals away from a kill and eaten carrion. For them eating was a matter of survival, not a philosophical, ethical, or moral decision. However, cereal grains were virtually absent from their diets.

Picture our history as a species—99% of it has been pre-agricultural. Agriculture remains the single most radical change in human history (even more radical than the internet) and resulted not only in changes in eating but in civilization and such associated changes as writing, economics, imperialism, government and religion. We have not caught up with these changes, and our bodies have not adapted to a diet based on grains. For about 150 years scientists have been aware of the "diseases of civilization" hypothesis. This is not new information, although it is not part of the orthodoxy of nutritionism. What has changed during the last fifty years is the incredibly rapid shift our society has made to a diet based almost exclusively on highly processed and refined foods that are designed for the healthy profits of the pharmaceutical-industrial food complex—not the health of the consumers who provide their profits. We must see this clearly. We are being exploited for profit in ways that are similar to the ways that animals raised on factory farms are being exploited for profit.

Eating may have an ethical dimension to it, but what you eat is not a statement of how virtuous or moral you are. What you eat does not make you holy or closer to God, virtuous, or "cool." What you eat and what you believe about what you eat, is shaped by your culture, your region, your budget, perhaps your religion, and what's available. While you might be trying to make the best possible food choices, your understanding of what constitutes "best" has been shaped by how you have been informed. If there are critical flaws in this information, and I believe that there are, then the conclusions you draw from you "know" will inevitably be flawed as well.

Many researchers have suspected a connection between a grain-based diet and the diseases of civilization, especially when the grains are combined and processed with poisons like carrageenan, soy, refined sugars, sugar substitutes and inedible waste products such as bran and soy lecithin. Many researchers have also pointed out that grains are not digested effectively by humans and that a process of fermentation takes place in the gut when these grains are introduced that produces gas and undigested residue.

Elaine Gottschall provides a good overview of the problems with grains and other complex carbohydrates in her book *Breaking the Vicious Cycle: Intestinal Health Through Diet*. She reviews scientific evidence about diet in the second chapter of this book and points out that in the early 1900s Dr. Christian Herter of Columbia University found that children who were losing weight and suffering from severe diarrhea always tolerated protein well, fats relatively well, and had bad reactions to carbohydrates. During the same time period specialists in children's diseases found that children with intestinal problems usually did not tolerate cow's milk or starchy carbohydrates such as grains, rice, corn, or potatoes. Several studies have illustrated a link between the high consumption of bread and sugar and both ulcerative colitis and Crohn's disease (1-10). Gottshall and others have speculated that poorly digested and fermenting residue from grain and sugars creates a bacterial overgrowth in the gut which triggers an auto-immune reaction in the inflammatory bowel disease sufferer. Gottschall's dietary plan is built upon the premise that by eliminating the foods that caused the bacterial overgrowth, the body will eventually return to a state of health. That's one of the reasons why the Specific Carbohydrate Diet is so strict. These bacteria only need a minute amount of complex carbohydrates on which to feed, so foods containing complex carbohydrates must be eliminated completely from the diet so that these unhealthy bacteria will be starved and thus killed off. In addition to grains, foods to avoid include sugars of all sorts— including refined sugars and milk sugars. Luckily milk sugars (lactose) can be broken down by some processing methods and so yogurt that is fermented for 24 hours (no commercial brands fit this, so you have to do it yourself) and most hard cheeses are allowed on the Specific Carbohydrate Diet. Unlike most other diets for IBD, this diet does not allow for potatoes.

> Gottschall points out that
> Unabsorbed carbohydrates constitute the most important source of gas in the intestine. For example, the lactose contained in one ounce of milk, if undigested and unabsorbed, will produce about 50 ml of gas in the intestine of normal people. But under abnormal conditions when

intestinal microbes have moved into the small intestine, the hydrogen gas production may be increased over one hundred-fold (17-18).

Gottschall goes on to argue that once the bacteria have started to increase in the small intestine, a vicious cycle begins with the ultimate result of inflammatory bowel disease.

Gottschall has done her research, and I recommend buying her book and reading it closely in order to understand why grains, most sugars, unprocessed milk products, starches, and fiber from grains are problematic. The key to foods being included or excluded from her diet plan is whether or not these foods contain disaccharides (double sugars). All animal fats and proteins are allowed on the diet as are most fruits and vegetables. Honey is also allowed since it is a simple carbohydrate. Gottschall has a very clear explanation of the problems that gluten causes for many people, and gluten's link to celiac disease. Some of her most interesting work involves suggesting links between problems with the gastrointestinal system and mental illnesses such as schizophrenia.

Perhaps the most critical connection she makes between the standard western diet and illness is its potential link to autism and the use of the Specific Carbohydrate Diet in treating autism. It's certainly interesting to note that diagnosed cases of autism among children have risen rapidly since the adoption of a diet based primarily on wheat, rice, corn, and soy.

As I've stated before, I followed the Specific Carbohydrate Diet strictly for two years, and it did help somewhat with my symptoms. Thousands of people swear by it and link long-term remission and the disappearance of symptoms to careful adherence to this diet. There is some research indicating that many children with autism who follow the Specific Carbohydrate Diet improve or recover completely. That discussion is beyond the scope of this book but should be pursued by anyone with a child diagnosed with autism.

Gastroenterologists generally don't see a link between diet and inflammatory bowel disease and so don't usually recommend the Specific Carbohydrate Diet as a treatment, but most of them don't discourage using it either. As always, should one decide to follow this diet, it should be done with the knowledge of your gastroenterologist, and you should not stop taking medications while following the diet. Most gastroenterologists will simply tell you that there haven't been any scientific studies of the Specific Carbohydrate Diet and so the claims are unfounded. This isn't really surprising since almost all clinical studies are funded by pharmaceutical companies, but this excuse about the Specific Carbohydrate Diet might be about to change. In March 2011 Rush University Medical Center began a clinical trial to test the effectiveness of the Specific Carbohydrate Diet in changing the population of bacteria/yeast in the gastrointestinal tract.

I try to avoid grains as much as possible, and I rarely eat bread, although I've found that I can eat small quantities of a few breads that didn't bother me. The problem is finding a commercially-produced bread that doesn't include soy, soy lecithin, carrageenan, or brown rice flour. Some local bakeries produce breads that fit these requirements, and one organic brand that I've found, Rudi's, also doesn't include these ingredients in some of its products. Still, I mostly avoid bread and products made of grain. I know that brown rice is one of the darlings of the natural food industry and of consumers who shop the natural foods stores, but two of my worst flares started after consuming brown rice at dinner parties where I didn't want to be "rude." I haven't eaten brown rice since I started using nicotine and my disease disappeared, and I don't plan to experiment on myself by trying it again. I'm also learning to say "no thank you."

Chapter 12
Alternative Approaches to Treating Inflammatory Bowel Disease

Like many of you reading this book, I explored a number of alternative treatments in attempting to deal with ulcerative colitis. In addition to traditional allopathic treatments such as steroids and immunomodulators, I explored naturopathy, acupuncture, and meditation. I also did yoga. I spent a year working with a naturopath and put so many foul-tasting teas into my system that I still have involuntary shudders at the thought of their bilge-water taste. I drank gallons of aloe vera and used poultices and oils in addition to other remedies. There are now several books available on naturopathic approaches to inflammatory bowel disease, and they seem to work for some people. Unfortunately, I didn't notice any improvement from these treatments. I also tried acupuncture on several occasions. Acupuncture was great for relieving the terrible pain I sometimes experienced in my joints and lower back (also symptoms of Inflammatory Bowel Disease), but the one time an acupuncturist worked on my IBD (without informing me in advance and without my permission) the flare I was experiencing actually got much worse.

What finally worked for me was nicotine. I'm not going to take on the anti-smoking forces—they are too large, too powerful, and too well-financed for that. I'm also not going to recommend that anyone begin using just any kind of tobacco products—that is a personal decision. However, I am going to point to my own experience and make it clear that nicotine has been a potent ally on my own journey from ulcerative colitis to health. I'll also point out that there is a strong body of scientific evidence indicating that nicotine provides some kind of protection from ulcerative colitis although the mechanism of this protection isn't yet known. By the way, the results are much less clear for Crohn's. Remember that tobacco is a plant, a natural product. I would *never* advocate that anyone start smoking commercially produced cigarettes or most any other tobacco product since these are absolutely drenched in harmful chemicals to "enhance" taste and burning rate, among other things. However, it is possible to find chemical-free, even organic, tobacco.

I have chosen to smoke organic, pesticide-free tobacco that is cured using the slow, natural, old-fashioned methods. This way my body is absorbing tobacco/nicotine and nothing else. By the way, if men can smoke (and I'll leave it up to you to decide whether or not that's sometimes appropriate), women can too. Even pipes! Your health and well-being are more important than arbitrary social convention.

I found it interesting to learn that many people develop ulcerative colitis or Crohn's disease after they quit smoking. It's unclear why this happens. Perhaps the nicotine has provided some kind of protective element, but no one really knows why people who quit smoking sometimes develop Inflammatory Bowel Disease. A number of studies have pointed to the protective qualities of nicotine for ulcerative colitis. Smokers have a lower incidence of the disease than non-smokers and many people experience the onset of ulcerative colitis after stopping smoking. Gastroenterologists are well-aware of the connection between nicotine and ulcerative colitis as well as that going back to smoking or using nicotine patches often brings on remission of the disease. A number of studies (none of them funded by the tobacco industry) have also demonstrated that nicotine is effective in putting ulcerative colitis into remission.

Crohn's alert: some research indicates that using nicotine may make Crohn's worse. My experiences with inflammation have been exclusively in the large intestine, although when I flared I also had ulcers in my mouth and developed ulcerative type sores on my skin. You probably should not use nicotine if your diagnosis is Crohn's, but, as always, make all treatment decisions under the supervision of your doctor. Kane notes, "we know that cigarette smokers are much more likely to develop Crohn's disease than nonsmokers and that cigarette smoking makes Crohn's disease worse."*

If you have ulcerative colitis and not Crohn's disease and want to engage in a doctor-supervised experiment with nicotine, the smoking cessation patches (transdermal nicotine) that are widely available might be a possible option. These patches deliver nicotine through the circulatory system without all of the added chemicals that come from cigarettes. I use these when I travel or when I'm in a situation where smoking is difficult. Like all of the medicines used to treat inflammatory bowel disease, nicotine has side effects. The short-term side effects include increased heart rate and blood flow to the heart as well as some temporary narrowing of the capillaries that carry the blood (while the nicotine is active). Some people who have used nicotine patches have reported vivid dreams, nervousness, and sweating. Nicotine can also focus mental concentration and help one relax. Some people who use patches have complained of dizziness, drowsiness, or nausea. Strong doses of nicotine taken orally (as in nicotine gum) may also cause hiccups or heartburn.

Making a decision about using nicotine is one that must be carefully considered. I've come across a number of posts on the internet from other ulcerative colitis sufferers who have made the decision to smoke or to use nicotine patches. It's really a matter of considering the trade-offs. Is it worth it to you suffer the symptoms of ulcerative colitis or the potential side effects of the medications used to treat it, to avoid the well-documented health risks of smoking? Is it more important to you to have a functioning colon and use nicotine than to have a colostomy? Only you and your doctor can make this decision for you. I made the decision to smoke a pipe. The health risks of smoking a pipe are much, much lower than the health risks for smoking cigarettes. I smoke organically grown, chemical-free tobacco. I decided that the quality of my life was more important than the possibility of losing some years at the end of my life. I smoke, I exercise, and I try to maintain a healthy lifestyle. I have never felt healthier or had more zest for life than I have now.

* Van der Heide F. Dijkstra A, Weersma RK, et al. Effects of active and passive smoking on disease course of Crohn's disease and ulcerative colitis. *InflammBowel Dis* 2009; 15 (8): 1199-2007. Retrieved from http://www.ncbi.nlm.nih.gov/pubmed/19170191

Chapter 13
Vitamins and Supplements

Vitamins and supplements need some consideration. One of the problems with inflammatory bowel disease (and other autoimmune diseases) is malnutrition, and so it's important to make sure that you get all the vitamins and minerals your body needs. If your digestive system is working properly, you should get most of what you need from what you eat—especially if you avoid vitamin-destroying foods such as cereals and grains, soy, and legumes. Just as with eating, I try to keep vitamins and supplements simple.

Many people with inflammatory bowel disease take fish oil capsules as a way of increasing their Omega-3 fatty acids. I've talked to people who swear that this has helped with their inflammatory bowel disease. I took fish oil capsules for a number of years, but I didn't see much impact on the course of my disease. I no longer take these—largely because I can't stand the taste when I belch them—and these invariably make me belch. Some fish oil capsules claim to eliminate this side effect. Since I didn't see much benefit from these, I haven't tried them. They might work for you, though, and are certainly worth a try if you can tolerate them.

Probiotics are also useful for many people. Probiotics are just foods or supplements that contain "good" bacteria to help in maintaining a healthy bacterial ecology in the digestive system. These probiotics can be found in food products such as yogurt, as well as in supplements. Look for high-quality, unsweetened yogurt and add your own honey, fruit, or stevia for sweetness if you wish. I took a powerful probiotic supplement for about six months while I was in a bad flare and didn't see much benefit. However, lots of people report good results from using these, and I do eat lots of homemade yogurt. I believe this helps maintain a good ecology in my digestive system.

I take three vitamins daily—Vitamin D, potassium, and a B-complex (which includes B12, B6, and folic acid). One of the most fascinating areas of research today has to do with Vitamin D and autoimmune diseases such as inflammatory bowel disease and multiple sclerosis. Almost everyone who develops one of these diseases turns out to have a vitamin D deficiency. This is probably why auto-immune diseases occur more frequently in temperate zones than in tropical zones. It could also explain why such diseases as multiple sclerosis occur with higher frequency in more northern latitudes. Historically humans get vitamin D through exposure to sunlight, but many of us no longer spend much time in the sun and if we do, we have sunscreen on and the sunscreen blocks the sun. Also, our species has moved away from the tropical regions where we evolved, and we now live all over the planet, a large percentage of us in climates for which we did not originally evolve. In short, we still need sun and sunlight. Most writers say that we need to get about twenty to thirty minutes of noon-day sun, daily. Many people are switching to full-spectrum light bulbs in their homes and offices in order to ward off depression and to increase healthy exposure to this essential spectrum of light.

I also take melatonin each night before bed. After a number of courses of corticosteroids, I've never been able to restore normal sleep patterns, and the melatonin helps me get to sleep and stay asleep. Lots of different claims are made for the health benefits of melatonin, including that it's good for our brains. That's not why I take it. It's a sleep aid for me.

Choose your vitamins and supplements very carefully. Quality is worth paying for here. Once more, it's important to read labels closely. For some reason, many vitamin products contain soy lecithin or soy. Many also contain artificial sweeteners—who knows why?

A final recommendation is to buy some powdered coconut and add this to your water. Coconut water is full of electrolytes and one serving only has about five calories. It's also a simple carbohydrate. I've also purchased the liquid form of coconut water and take packets of this with me when I travel. I also drink this for a quick pick-me-up.

Chapter 14
My Version of a Diet for Inflammatory Bowel Disease: Keeping It Simple

I've talked a lot about food and dietary choices in this book, but I'd like to use this chapter to talk about what I eat—what has worked for me on this journey and what I find I have to avoid. I also want to once more make the point that our food choices are not about morality, and we do not become virtuous or evil people because of the foods we consume. Too often we are made to feel guilty about what we eat. Unfortunately, attempts to follow the rules of dietary correctness that have become so powerful in western culture often damage the health and ecology of our bodies. I also want to emphasize the importance of not giving oneself a hard time if a dietary slip occurs. It can be very difficult to follow any diet while traveling, eating in a restaurant, or eating at other people's houses. I do the best I can and accept that in the food ecology of today, there will be occasional slips.

For two years I strictly followed the Specific Carbohydrate Diet. I believe this diet helped correct the ecological imbalances in my gut and my body. However, this diet can be very restrictive, and now that I am healthy I find that I can follow many of its basic guidelines but can also tolerate some of the foods it forbids. I've also found that some foods it allows don't work well for me. I've modified the diet quite a bit. Most of these modifications have come from the reading I've done on human evolution and on the diet that humans consumed through the vast majority of our history. We need to eat the diet our bodies evolved to eat, and that means keeping things pretty simple and staying away from the processed "foods" produced by the food industry. It's absolutely critical to read labels closely and to eat foods that don't contain chemical additives, added fiber, added sugar, and soy. This applies to "natural" and "organic" products too.

We don't use processed foods. That means that we prepare and cook all of our foods ourselves. It takes more time than using processed foods, but the benefits are incalculable. Mostly I eat meats, a variety of well-cooked vegetables, fresh fruits and berries, homemade yogurt, cheese, nuts, and most spices and chiles. I've found that potatoes and white rice don't seem to bother me as long as I don't overdo them, and I can eat some corn products, although I never eat corn kernels or popcorn. I can eat hominy in limited amounts (usually prepared as posole), corn tortillas (without additives), and even cornbread, as long as I don't over-indulge. I even eat a bit of dark chocolate sometimes. For sweeteners I usually use honey or stevia, although I'll eat a bit of sugar sometimes when I'm traveling or visiting someone. I avoided coffee for years, but now that I'm healthy it doesn't seem to bother me, and I enjoy several cups of coffee every day. While I was getting healthier, I drank cold-pressed coffee for a time. This coffee is less acidic than regular coffee, and it allowed me to reintroduce coffee to my system. Since I've been fully healthy, coffee has not bothered me. I drink lots of black and green tea as well as herbal teas such as chamomile. I also drink a lot of coconut water and regular water.

Avoiding certain foods, and especially additives, is what has truly allowed me to move forward on my journey toward health. Some foods bother me more than others, even if they're fresh. Usually if a food causes me to burp or pass gas, I know that it's a food that I need to avoid. I have a hard time with raw vegetables, and lettuce always makes me sick, so I avoid these. Fiber-heavy foods cause problems for me. One real culprit in the past has been brown rice, so I even avoid foods that have brown rice flour as an ingredient. Beans and legumes are among the darlings of the natural food industry, and are allowed, with caution, on the Specific Carbohydrate Diet, but beans are very difficult for humans to digest. I used to eat beans of various sorts on an almost daily basis, but I avoid them now (with the exception of well-cooked green beans).

I try to eat a low fiber diet, and that's one of the reasons I make sure my vegetables are cooked well. This helps break down the fiber they contain. Even so, leafy vegetables such as spinach will often turn up undigested in the toilet bowl if I eat them, so I try to keep my consumption of them low. This can be an issue if you eat too much raw fruit as well. Of course, there's also the issue of fructose (another sugar) if you eat too much fruit of any kind.

I don't eat cereals and grains—not even the gluten free versions—for the most part, although there are occasions (traveling or eating at people's houses) where I will eat a piece of bread or a biscuit. Small amounts of grain don't cause real problems for me. The bigger problem is the additives. It's almost impossible to find commercially produced bread that doesn't include soy and sugar although some organic brands offer good choices. Ezekiel bread, although popular among many, contains soy, so I avoid this.

I also drink very little. I stopped using alcohol when I was taking 6mp, and I've never really felt much desire to go back to it. Alcohol is almost always made from grains and it also contains lots of sugar.

I do my best to avoid soy and soy products such as soy lecithin. I also try to keep my fiber intake as low as possible and would never eat any product that contained bran. Bran is nothing more than industrial waste and is really not fit for human consumption.

Dairy products are problematical. I never drink milk, but I do use heavy (table) cream or half and half in coffee and cooking, and this doesn't bother me. Table cream is essentially fat and doesn't contain lactose (a form of sugar), which is what causes problems for me. We make our own yogurt and ferment it for 24 hours so that all of the lactose is broken down. Most hard cheeses don't contain lactose either, so I eat them without worries.

The one thing I never allow to pass my lips is carrageenan. Remember, researchers use carrageenan to induce inflammatory bowel disease in lab animals. That's one of the reasons I read labels so conscientiously and one of the reasons I'm careful to avoid commercially-produced dairy products. Almost all versions of whipping cream and half and half contain carrageenan, so if you decide to try these, make sure there's no carrageenan added. The same applies to almost all products such as ice cream or puddings. Carrageenan will pop up in the most unexpected places, so keep your eye out for this destructive product.

I try to be flexible in my eating and get as much variety as possible. I don't view eating from a moral or ethical perspective—it's about my health not my virtue or goodness. If I slip up or accidentally eat something I normally avoid, I just accept it and move on. Above all, I try to enjoy what I eat and to approach my food with pleasure and gratitude.

Chapter 15
Growing a Healthy Mind

Just as I've discussed medicine and nutrition as ecologies, I'd like to consider ourselves as ecologies, and this means including our thinking and our mental habits. One of the tragedies of western thinking has been the tendency to view the body and the mind (or spirit) as separate from each other. When this happens, we typically view the body as of lesser importance than the mind or spirit. Even worse, we often view our bodies as little more than machines that needs repairs and replacement parts. This mechanistic vision of the body denies the body its connectedness and creates a divided vision in which the body is severed from the mind or spirit. Too often the body becomes a scapegoat that can be blamed for not working as it should or for bringing pain and suffering to us. Of course, often when the body isn't working correctly, the mind isn't functioning at its highest level either. Just like our bodies, our minds are products of our evolution. We are whole beings, not divided beings, and one of the most important steps we can make is to forgive ourselves for the pain and suffering we have experienced. Blame does not serve your healing. Neither do suffering and sacrifice. They weaken you and make you unable to be your best self—the best parent, spouse, colleague, or friend that you can be. Blame, resentment, suffering, and victimhood—dwelling in the past, in old mistakes and wrongs—all of these need to be removed from the ecology of our body and spirit, silenced in our minds, and replaced with an open, forgiving, accepting, and optimistic attitude. The healing process is not just a physical process; it's also a mental one, and the most important steps toward healing begin with forgiveness and acceptance. Gratitude is also key to the healing process. Nothing heals more than taking stock of our situation and realizing just how many things we have to be grateful for—even in the darkest of times.

I'm not claiming that positive thinking or a happy attitude will cure inflammatory bowel disease although it will help you get through each day and might even help the healing process. I am going to argue that gratitude and happiness can help us approach each day with a sense of anticipation rather than dread and help us to move forward with our lives in spite of suffering. One of the worst things about inflammatory bowel disease is that it often leads to depression, even despair, as we anticipate and dread the difficulties the disease poses. It's hard to be joyful when you're watching a toilet fill with blood for the twentieth time in a single day. Keep reminding yourself that you have the right to define yourself and that you are not defined by disease. It is essential to claim your own self and identity independently of any illness you might be experiencing.

There's something to be said for the old cliché, "Laughter is the best medicine." If you can laugh at inflammatory bowel disease, each day will become easier to get through. The eighteenth century British writer, Horace Walpole, once wrote, "Life is a tragedy for those who feel, but a comedy to those who think," and he's right. To laugh we need to have an element of detachment, of separation, and this can be important not just for laughter, but for helping us to observe what's going on with our bodies. In the chapter, "Solitude," from *Walden*, Henry David Thoreau talks about our ability to separate ourselves from whatever situation we find ourselves participating in and instead to observe both the situation and ourselves within the situation. This stepping back and becoming the observer can help us achieve the detachment that we need to notice what is really happening with our bodies and also to realize that we are much more than the body. It's hard to stress just how much the ability to step back and observe ourselves can help us regain some control over a situation rather than feeling as though we're being pulled down into a spinning vortex without any control at all.

Poets in the twentieth century, such as Gary Snyder or Robinson Jeffers, as well as spiritual writers such as Eckhart Tolle, emphasize the necessity of "presence." These writers all point to the crucial importance of simply paying attention, of being present for our life and observing it. This might be called mindfulness. When we practice "presence" or "mindfulness," we are doing nothing more than trying to stay in this moment and to be aware of what is happening at this moment rather than living in the past or anticipating the future. After all, this moment is all we have. This habit of mind can help us escape worry, and all of us know that worrying about things is like a child riding a rocking horse—it doesn't take us anywhere and we end up feeling rattled. Being present for the actual moments of our life instead of living in the past or the future can help open our awareness and bring a sense of calm and even understanding. Try spending a few moments now observing what's happening in your mind. What do you notice? Many times the first thing to surface is anxiety, and that's not surprising. We've developed some poor habits of unhelpful places where our minds will rush to take us if we're not careful. Anxiety accompanies inflammatory bowel disease, but it can be useful to observe this anxiety and then try to deal with it. Perhaps you could try just breathing deeply while being conscious of the breath flowing in and out as you visualize the anxiety melting into a pool of light. Can you picture it in your imagination? Can you picture the anxiety melting, or even dissolving into dust that just blows away. Maybe it is being replaced by light made up of greens and golds; maybe it is becoming a soft breeze that soothes and relaxes.

A good way to practice presence is to continue the process of observation. Try becoming aware of your body. Start with your fingers or toes and focus your awareness there. Try focusing your awareness on your stomach, your intestines, your colon. Can you visualize something positive and healing replacing the disease? I like to visualize a healing, golden honey flowing through my digestive system and replacing any diseased tissue with healthy tissue. I actually learned about this technique from my brother-in-law who, 25 years ago, visualized the potent chemotherapy drug entering his body as a healing and soothing honey. He became ill only on the first day of the chemotherapy treatment. He's been well ever since.

One of the best things detachment and presence can provide is the ability to observe the repetitive refrains that run through our minds. Often these are built around past experiences or the anticipation of what the future might hold. If you're able to observe the words that keep running through your mind, try to discover if these are positive or negative. If the thoughts are negative, they're probably a source of stress or anxiety. Bring your mind back to the present moment and seek out the good in it. What about thoughts of the future? Sometimes we do have to plan and make sure we know pieces of information such as the location of bathrooms, but do you find yourself saying things like, "I'm falling apart," or "I don't know what I'm going to do," over and over and over in your mind? Replacing statements such as these with phrases like, "I feel better and better, " or "I feel good," or "I have more energy," might not heal your disease, but they might make you feel better and help you to approach each day with a more positive outlook, and that can't hurt. It's definitely a lot better than adding one more drug to the cocktail you're probably already putting into your system.

Other practices that people have found helpful are meditation and yoga. Meditation is a way of achieving presence, but, more crucially, it helps us achieve a state of calm and relieves stress. It can also help us achieve more awareness of our bodies and what is happening in them. Our bodies do speak to us, but we need to learn to listen. Yoga also helps achieve body-awareness and for many people yoga is also a good way to work toward being more present and aware of the moment.

I find it useful to try to connect to the natural world, and I'm lucky since I live in an area that's beautiful and somewhat rural. Even the most urbanized environment provides opportunities to connect with other living and growing things such as plants or pets. Gardening, even keeping an herb garden or growing tomato plants if you live in an apartment, is a great way to connect with things outside ourselves that are growing in a healthy way. If you're able to garden outside this will also help increase your vitamin D. Low levels of this crucial vitamin are increasingly being linked by researchers to a whole range of auto-immune diseases. Anyone who does not live in a tropical or subtropical environment should look into taking vitamin D every day.

A tool that many people are finding effective in dealing with trauma, anxiety, and illness is called "emotional freedom technique," or EFT for short. If one has experienced a big loss or trauma, EFT would be a great tool to explore, and information about EFT is widely available on the internet—including many demonstrations of the technique on Youtube. EFT involves "tapping" on specified acupuncture points in order to "rewire" the brain. The idea is that when an individual experiences trauma, the wiring of the brain was changed. The trauma can be retriggered and relived over and over again because the neural pathways of the trauma are now in place, wired into the brain. "Trauma" is another word for "trance." When the trauma is triggered, for example, by seeing an image of the Twin Towers of the World Trade Center falling or by something more personal such as bright red blood in the toilet, trance is induced. Traditional forms of psychotherapy such as talk therapy do not impact this "wiring," but EFT techniques, according to a number of studies, can permanently change brain patterns and lead to the overcoming of phobias, anxiety, destructive habits, and even physical pain. It's simple to self-administer, quick to learn, and easy to master. It not only is proving to be highly effective, it's free. Some practitioners report success in using EFT with auto-immune diseases such as multiple sclerosis. Check out some of these sites for further discussion, instruction, demonstrations, and testimonials:

  www.eftuniverse.com
  www.emofree.com
  www.youtube.com/watch?v=dYhYp3lzlX8
  www.eft-for-transformation.com/eft-gary-craig.html
  www.masteringeft.com
  www.thetappingsolution.com

 There's even a documentary film about EFT available entitled, "Try It on Everything." There is no downside or negative effect from the use of EFT, so it can't hurt—it can only help. EFT, and related modalities such as TFT (Thought Field Therapy) and TAT (Tapas Acupressure Technique) might well revolutionize not only the fields of psychotherapy and the treatment of post-traumatic stress, but may soon be considered the central "go to" techniques of preventive care and alternative healing.

 Any kind of pain can turn us inward toward focusing almost exclusively on ourselves and our personal discomfort. As Emily Dickinson pointed out, "Pain has an element of blank." It's crucially important that we find ways to move outside of ourselves and not to become obsessed with our illness. I often think of the way Ben Franklin began and ended each day. Each morning his question for himself was, "What good will I do today?' Each night he asked himself, "What good have I done today?" It's hard to imagine a better prayer or a better way of escaping what can often seem like the prison of illness and even the prison of the self and of self-absorption.

 Each of you will have to find what works best for you as an individual, but try to find ways to avoid stress and worry. These aren't productive and can exacerbate a flare. I've certainly had flares start as a result of stress in the past, and I'm sure this is also a familiar pattern for many readers. Try to achieve some level of detachment and as much "presence" as you can. It can only help.

Chapter 16
Revisioning Illness

I've been thinking about language all of my life. One of the things that has become more and more clear as linguists, psychologists, and philosophers have investigated language is the role language plays in how we think about, and even create, reality through the words we use. Some of the most exciting discoveries about the way the human mind works in recent years have come from the field of cognitive linguistics and the work of such writers as George Lakoff, Mark Johnson, and Steven Pinker. I'm only going to give a brief overview of this topic here, but if you're interested (and I hope you will be), I've listed some of the most important contributions to this field in the "Sources" section.

One thing all of these writers agree on is that our minds work to build a vision of the "real" world, of "what is," through the process of metaphor. Language itself works through metaphor, and our way of thinking is deeply metaphorical. Metaphor is how we construct the world or at least the reality that we think of as the world. It's also how we know this reality and how we envision it in our minds. We can "slam" a ball or "dodge" the issue. We get "up" in the morning, and we can "greet the day" or "embrace the future." Metaphor is really a pretty simple concept. The word comes from the Greek word, *metaphoros*. When Ellen and I took our honeymoon and visited her family in Greece, I got really excited when I saw a truck with the word *metaphoros* on the side of it and thought what a poetic culture the Greeks had. I pointed it out to Ellen, and she said,

"Oh, that's a moving van." That's exactly how metaphor works. It moves a concept from one place (a place of origin—usually called the "source") to another place (the receiver—usually called the "target"). How many times have you thought about how you need to "conquer" Crohn's or ulcerative colitis? There's an example of a metaphor. When you're thinking in this way, you've essentially started thinking of your disease in terms of a war. Is that the best way to visualize this auto-immune disease? Do you really want to be at war with yourself?

I'm not suggesting a simplistic "change your thinking, change your life" approach to considering inflammatory bowel disease and your relationship to this disease. The way we conceive of the world, the way we envision the world, the way we create thought patterns through the words we use has real impacts on our health and our relationship with our body. What I'm pointing out is that you can "revision" the way you use words when you think about and talk about inflammatory bowel disease. Like everything else, language is a system, an ecology. During the last 25 years, cognitive linguists have opened up new ways of understanding the interactions between the mind and language. I'm absolutely certain that how we think and the words we select to shape our thinking have an impact on our health.

One of the ways to think about the metaphors we use every day is to think of them as different topics or areas of meaning (linguists refer to these as metaphoric gestalts or metaphoric domains). Here are some examples. When we talk about love and relationships we often talk about them in terms of a journey, in terms of moving forward or backward or even standing still. Have you ever heard anyone say (or said yourself), "this relationship has hit a dead end"? When we talk about arguments or disagreements, we often talk in terms of war or weapons. "I demolished his arguments." "She has a cutting tongue." These metaphoric areas of meaning help "frame" the way we think about such things as illness. When thinking about what "framing" an issue is, think about it in terms of taking a photograph. Anytime we take a photograph, we include some things (in the frame) and exclude others. If something is inside the frame, it's part of the discussion, and the words we use create the way an issue is framed or thought about. If it's out of the frame, we probably won't be thinking about it at all, yet issues and ideas outside of our snapshot can be important too.

Spend a minute thinking about who it is that you spend the most time talking with each day. Your mom? Your best friend? You might argue with this person as well. The truth is that you spend the most time in conversation with yourself. All of us have a running conversation with ourselves going almost all the time—often even when we're talking with someone else. Are there ways in which this ongoing conversation with ourselves (as well as with others) constructs the way we think about the disease we are "struggling" with?

Spend another moment thinking about the words you use when you think about the digestive health problems you've experienced. One of the more interesting topic areas I've noticed in relationship to inflammatory bowel disease is the set of metaphors that are drawn from the world of bureaucracy. Have you and your physician ever discussed ways to "manage" your disease? It's most fitting for the auto-immune diseases that are increasing so rapidly for our doctors to define their roles as a boss who "manages" a variety of body parts, of systems and trying to get them to "cooperate" or "work together smoothly." Have you ever heard a colonoscopy or sigmoidoscopy defined as a "procedure"—how about the removal of an essential body part as a "procedure"? Do we see the disease as a "process," a process that can be managed or mitigated? I, personally, don't like the image of my gastroenterologist as a mid-level manager, a bureaucrat whose primary goal is efficiency and keeping problems to a minimum. He's too smart for that. I prefer metaphors of partnership and teamwork. It's appropriate for the age we dwell in that these images would emerge as central just as the nature of the disease as "chronic," lifelong, something that can't be cured but can be managed is appropriate for our age.

Think of what "chronic" implies. The word "chronic," like so many scientific terms, comes from Greek. "Chronos" was the personification (god) of time, and from his name we get words such as "chronology" which means the order of events in time. Officially there is no cure for a chronic disease—it's one that we're stuck with for the rest of our life.

Thinking about illness in connection with the language used to talk about it opens new insights into our relationship with illness. Consider the ways we've thought of diseases in the past. In the nineteenth century tuberculosis was the disease that drew the most attention, and tuberculosis was generally referred to as "consumption." The vision of the disease was one that consumed the sufferer from the inside, a disease in which the sufferer wasted away. In the twentieth century cancer began to command the public's attention (and still does). The word "cancer" comes from the Greek word for "crab" and is generally conceived of as an alien invader attacking the body.

Auto-immune diseases are the diseases of the twenty-first century. These diseases are built around images of betrayal, of treason. In auto-immune diseases the body attacks itself. In this constellation of diseases the body's defense system becomes the attacker, and the sufferer is subjected to constant "friendly fire" from what should be an ally. The attack of the body by the body invariably creates a sense of the body as traitor, as betrayer, and ultimately leads to a vision of the body and of ourselves as alienated, separated. Even worse, this disease is seen as chronic, as something that will be present to the end of the sufferer's life. A state of illness comes to define "normality" for the sufferer—this is what one expects life to be like. Auto-immune diseases can't be overcome, but only "managed." The only possible cure is to cut the offender out of the body, to remove it completely. These diseases are also viewed as a process of degeneration in which the only expectation the sufferer really has is of becoming worse. I can't imagine a more powerful way to prevent one from healing than to view disease as normal, as the expected way of living.

I can't give you the right words or metaphors to use when you think about illness, but I can suggest that you try to find positive metaphors that will reinforce the healing process and create a sense of you—not the disease—as being in control.

You are not a disease.

Readings and Sources

Allan, Christian B. and Lutz, Wolfgang. *Life Without Bread: How a Low-Carbohydrate Diet Can Save Your Life.* New York: McGraw Hill, 2000.

Appleton, Nancy and Jacobs, G.N. *Suicide by Sugar: A Startling Look at Our #1 National Addiction.* Square One Publishers, 2009. This book has some good information about sugar, but the authors identify this as essentially the main problem with our diet. Otherwise they follow standard diet recommendations.

Banks, P.A., Present, D.H. and Steiner, P. *The Crohn's Disease and Ulcerative Colitis Fact Book.* National Foundation for Ileitis & Colitis. New York: Charles Scribner's Sons, 1983. Dated but often recommended by gastroenterologists.

Bernstein, Richard K. *Dr. Bernstein's Diabetes Solution: The Complete Guide to Achieving Normal Blood Sugars.* New York: Little, Brown and Company, 2007.

Black, J. and Cummings D. *Living With Crohn's & Colitis: A Comprehensive Naturopathic Guide for Complete Digestive Wellness.* Hatherleigh Press, 2010. It's hard to recommend this book; it's a naturopathic guide that does have some interesting information about "tapping" or the emotional freedom technique (EFT).

Cordain, Loren. *The Paleo-Diet: Lose Weight and Get Healthy by Eating the Food You Were Designed to Eat.* Hoboken, NJ: John Wiley and Sons, 2002.

Dahlman, D. *Why Doesn't My Doctor Know This? Conquering Irritable Bowel Syndrome, Inflammatory Bowel Disease, Crohn's Disease and Colitis.* Garden City, NY. Madeasy publishing, 2008. I can't recommend this; he also sees IBD as the end result of irritable bowel syndrome and IBS is essentially what this book is about. He also wants to "cure" by selling you lots of supplements.

De Vany, Arthur. *The New Evolution Diet: What Our Paleolithic Ancestors Can Teach Us about Weight Loss, Fitness, and Aging.* Rodale Books, 2010. This book has some interesting insights but isn't really aimed at Inflammatory Bowel Disease.

Gibbons, D. L., *The Self-Help Way to Treat Colitis and Other IBS Conditions* (2nd edition). New York: McGraw Hill (2001). Interesting observations about the medical community and drug corporations but some advice I'd stay far away from such as refined white bread and refined sugar as being IBD friendly foods; he also sees IBD as little more than a severe form of irritable bowel syndrome.

Gottschall, Elaine. *Breaking the Vicious Cycle: Intestinal Health Through Diet.* Baltimore: The Kirkton Press, 2010. This is the key book for the Specific Carbohydrate Diet. It's filled with useful and unusual insights.

Groves, Barry. *Trick and Treat: How 'Healthy Eating' is Making Us Ill.* London: Hammersmith Press. 2008. I highly recommend this for an analysis of the standard diet and the problems with this diet.

Hare, S. *How to Beat Ulcerative Colitis Naturally.* Stewart Hare, 2011. Don't waste your money. Hare lists some of the natural things such as aloe vera that are reputed to help with IBD but this SHORT collection doesn't even approach being a pamphlet.

Kalibjian, C. *Straight From the Gut: Living with Crohn's Disease & Ulcerative Colitis.* Sebastopol, CA: O'Reilly & Associates, 2003.

Kane, Sunanda V. *IBD Self-Management: The AGA Guide to Crohn's Disease and Ulcerative Colitis.* Bethesda, MD: AGA Press. 2010. print. This is a good straightforward presentation of Inflammatory Bowel Disease and strategies for living with this disease. Kane takes a common sense approach and emphasizes the importance of the patient taking control of the disease and managing the disease. She provides a clear description of the disease and has some good advice on diet.

Klein, D. *Self Healing: Colitis & Crohn's: The Complete Wholistic Guide to Healing the Gut & Staying Well.* (3rd edition). Sebastopol, CA: Colitis & Crohn's Health Recovery

Center, 2009. Can't recommend this. The author advocates a vegan diet and fiber.

Knoepp, Werner L. 2011. "The National Sugar Epidemic Is Killing Us: America's Sugar Consumption At Lethal Levels. Web page. http://www.website-articles- net/Art/293/327/The-National-Sugar-Epidemic-Is-Killing-Us-America-s-Sugar-Consumption-At-Lethal-Levels.html

Lakoff, George and Johnson, Mark. *Metaphors We Live By.* Chicago: The University of Chicago Press. 1980, 2003.

Land, Linda. *The Gift of Remission: A Journey into Multiple Sclerosis and Back Again-Prevent, Stop and Recover from Autoimmune Disease.* Outskirts Press, 2009.

Lang, J. M. *Learning Sickness: A Year with Crohn's Disease.* Sterling, VA., Capital Books, 2004. Learning to cope with Inflammatory Bowel Disease.

Monastyrsky, K. *Fiber Menace: The Truth About Fiber's Role in Diet Failure, Constipation, Hemorrhoids, Irritable Bowel Syndrome, Ulcerative Colitis, Crohn's Disease, and Colon Cancer.* U.S. Ageless Press, 2008.

Pinker, Steven. *How the Mind Works.* New York: W. W. Norton, 2009. Kindle edition.

Pinker, Steven, *The Stuff of Thought: Language As a Window into Human Nature.* New York: Viking Penguin, 2007.

Pollan, Michael. *In Defense of Food: An Eater's Manifesto.* NY: Penguin 2008-2009. I highly recommend this for an analysis of the standard diet and some of the problems with it.

Pollan, Michael. *The Omnivore's Dilemma: A Natural History of Four Meals*. New York: Penguin, 2007.

Ponting, Clive. *A New Green History of the World: The Environment and the Collapse of Great Civilizations*. New York: Penguin Books, 2007.

Sklar, Jill. *The First Year: Crohn's Disease and Ulcerative Colitis: A Patient-Expert Walks You Through Everything you need to Learn and Do.* (2nd edition). New York: Da Capo Press, 2007. Useful but Kane and Warner& Barto are better—does have advice on how to cope with the disease.

Sontag, Susan. *Illness as Metaphor and AIDS and Its Metaphors*. New York: St Martin's Press: 1977, 1988 (1990).

Taubes, Gary. *Good Calories, Bad Calories: Challenging the Conventional Wisdom on Diet, Weight Control, and Disease*. New York: Alfred A. Knopf, 2007. This book is essential to understanding problems with the current orthodoxy about food and health as well as the problems with the science behind current nutritional thinking.

Taubes, Gary. *Why We Get Fat and What to Do about It*. New York: Alfred A. Knopf, 2011.This is a more accessible doorway to many of Taubes' insights.

Tubesing, A. *ColitiScope: Living With Crohn's Disease and Ulcerative Colitis: Adventures, Humor, Insights*. Albuquerque, NM, 2009. A fun account of living with the disease.

Warner, A.S. and Barto, A.E. *100 Questions and Answers about Crohn's Disease and Ulcerative Colitis: A Lahey Clinic Guide* (2nd edition). Sudbury, Mass: Jones and Bartlett (2010); Mobipocket.com 2010. Kindle edition. This is another good resource.

ABOUT THE AUTHOR

Larry K. Hartsfield is a professor of English and Environmental Studies at Fort Lewis College in Durango, Colorado. He earned his Ph.D. in American Civilization at the University of Texas at Austin. He is also the author of *The American Response to Professional Crime: 1870-1917*.

Printed in Poland
by Amazon Fulfillment
Poland Sp. z o.o., Wrocław